I Am Just Me

My Life with Dyslexia and Dysgraphia

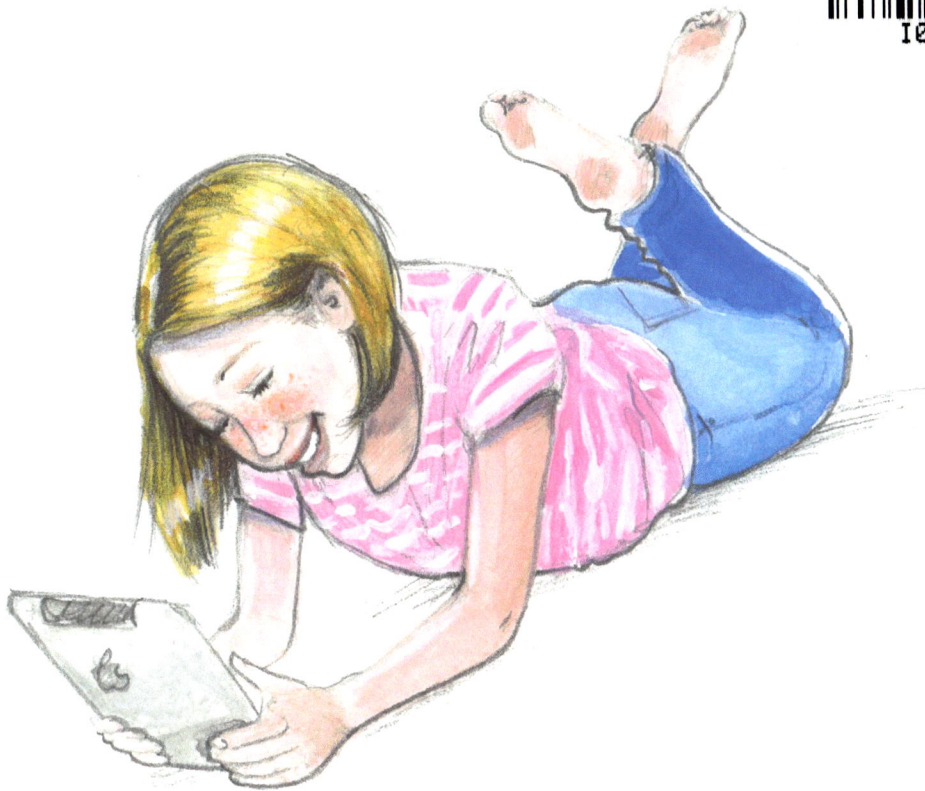

Sky Burke
and Penny Weber
illustrated by Penny Weber

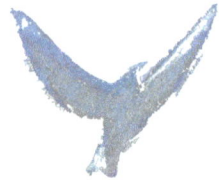

Thank you Sky for your courage and inspiration.
-Penny Weber

This book is for all the kids who are different and the people who appreciate others' differences.

I dedicate this book to my dad Kenneth F. Burke Jr. I know he is always watching over me and is forever in my heart. I love you to the moon and stars and back again.

I am so thankful for my creative and talented neighbor, illustrator, and co-author Penny Weber who made this book happen.

Thank you Aunt Lhea Scotto-Laub for writing my bio and Sarah Dillon for taking my headshots. To Bridget Cariello, Regional Coordinator for the Self-Advocacy Association of New York State for giving me a place for my voice to be heard.

Thank you to all of my past, present, and future teachers. Thank you to all the teachers that have made a difference in the life of a child who has a disability and truly understand the gifts they have to offer to the world.

I am grateful to Smart Kids with Learning Disabilities for the Fred J Epstein Award Youth Achievement Award and recognizing me as a "smart kid with a learning disability."

Thank you to the Long Island Advocacy Center for teaching my mom her rights, effective advocacy skills, and my rights as an individual with a disability that she in return shared with me. This was the most empowering gift I have ever received.

Special thanks to my amazing family: my new dad Pete, who stays up late nights to help me with my homework, my big sister Aurora who is always there for me and inspires me everyday by example, my brother Bailey who always puts a smile on my face and reminds me often that Autism is a gift to the world, my sister Skylar who always has bright creative ideas and works hard everyday to overcome her own obstacles, and my sister Bailey who is an exceptional leader that supports self-advocacy and spreading the word about disability awareness.

There are no words to thank my mom Beverly who supports me in every direction I go and who is the best momanger EVER!
-Sky Burke

This book is the beautiful story of a girl whose spirit soared, despite all of the challenges she faced. Sky's story is inspiring and uplifting – particularly for children who are beginning their journey of self-advocacy. Every child needs examples to inspire hope and optimism; Sky's story teaches all of us – adult and child alike – to know and accept ourselves, and to find our own voices. Parents, teachers, and children can all learn much from Sky's example and the advice her mother shares.
~Cara M. English, MA, Licensed Associate Counselor, Doctor of Behavioral Health Candidate
~Tempe, AZ

This book is truly remarkable and will change the way students with Learning Disabilities view themselves and empower them to advocate for their own needs. This book has the ability to modernize assistive technology for students with dyslexia and dysgraphia in school, which is way overdue. A must read for all students who feel different or left out. Sky Burke is Limitless
~Rachelle D. Sokul, Esq., a Lawyer with Dyslexia ~Queens, NY

Sky's strong leadership is well beyond her years. She is a bright young girl who will go places! I wish her the best of luck in all she does! Cathy Loquercio
~Self Advocate and President of the Self Advocacy Association Of New York State

We think it was brave of Sky to share her story, so others can learn from it. It was a very inspiring book. Great story!
~Mrs. Menechino's 1st grade Class, Merrimac Elementary School 2012-2013 ~Holbrook, NY

In Early Childhood, we tell children they can change the world. Sky's story is evidence of this truth. She has shown us that not only can a child change her own world through self-advocacy, but by sharing her story she empowers others to do the same. Parents, students and educators will benefit by hearing Sky's powerful message to listen to children because a child who is included in her educational journey will become a successful learner.
~Judi Fouchet, School Board Member and Early Childhood Provider ~Southold, NY

Professional athletes, movies stars, and celebrities do NOT inspire me. Children inspire me. Sky Burke is one of those children. I often think when I am speaking to children if they only knew how powerful they were and how quickly they could reach and inspire their peers. Sky Burke knows who she is. This book is not just for children it is for everyone. Read it and let the child in you become inspired by the spirit in Sky!!
David J. Flood , Youth Inspirational Speaker~ www.davidjflood.com ~Northport, NY

An inspiring story about a brave little girl who refuses to be defined or confined by a diagnosis
~April Velasco, PhD, Psychologist ~NY, NY

Wow! What an amazing and brave girl Sky is. For her to turn the difficulties that troubled her most in life and write a book about it shows true commitment to her education! It is a great way to help other children learn to step up and take charge of their disability and life. I wish I had more students who try as hard as Sky does. The fact that she wants to be treated like the other kids and strives for nothing less, speaks volumes of her persistence and personality. The book has a great moral, when a mountain is put in your path; find a way to climb over it! Don't let your disability define you, let it improve you and reach for the Sky!
~Kristine Jarnich, Texas Certified Teacher. Amarillo, Tx.

When Beverly and Sky gave me the honor of reviewing this book, I had (happy) tears in my eyes before I finished Sky's dedications. As a parent of a child with learning disabilities and a professional in the field of special education this story gives me hope that our worlds will continue to change for the better! Sky Burke, you are an inspiration to every child, young adult and educational professional. I have a feeling this is only the first of many informative stories we will read about you and your journey! Thank you for letting me be part of that journey.

~Helene Fallon, Project Coordinator, Long Island Parent Center, Center for Community Inclusion, Adjunct Faculty, Long Island University, Long Island Advocacy Center Regional Partner, Parent Training Information Center

Whose words these are I think I know,
the students need Sky in the village though
Dyslexia/Dysgraphia will not see her stopping here,
to watch assistive technology fill up with kids

Sky's words are lovely, bright, and real,
She has advocacy to keep
and miles to go before she teach,
and miles to go before she reach
-inspired by Robert Frost (Stopping by the Woods on a Snowy Evening) and Sky Burke (I Am Just Me)
-Sky you are truly inspirational and will open the bright blue sky
to others in need!!! Sedulous!!! ~Janine Caltabellotta, Parent and Reading teacher

I have had the opportunity to be on the sidelines, or better, to orbit in Sky's galaxy during this time. I have watched Sky's transformation from a young, shy, intimidated, little girl who believed all of the wrong things about herself, into a young girl who has strength, courage and an immense understanding of who she is. Sky's ability to use supports and technology to let her strengths shine through and to be able to share what works for her has changed her future. I am very thankful to have had the privilege of learning from my dear friend, Beverly, Sky's mother. Her belief in her children and all of our children, and her consistent message to help parents listen, love, and support and encourage our children, helps to change the life outcomes of so many families. She reminds me to focus and celebrate our children's strength's daily, while balancing our "momanager". She has moved heaven and earth for her children.
This is a blessed family who's Sky has no limit!
Valerie DeClara, Advocate and parent ~Ocenside NY

Forward

I once read somewhere that if you divide the sky into 27 million parts that each of those 27 million parts would contain not just stars but entire galaxies. Sitting down to write, I am reflecting on the infinite possibilities of life and the many stars that shine brightly in it. My first thought is of a widely known Self-Advocacy favorite written by Steve Holmes, " David's Song" or "We Are All Shining Stars", as the self-advocates would sometimes call it. Research says there is an estimated sextillion stars (only about 200 billion in our little galaxy). The thing about stars is that they are like snowflakes. Each one is different; each one is uniquely and delicately designed from creative energies and life force. This is the story of self-advocacy. This is the story of Sky.

I first heard of Sky Burke through a mutual colleague and immediately thought she would make a nice addition to our "Youth Team" at The Self-Advocacy Association of NYS. Though a meteoroid is significantly smaller than an asteroid, its visible streaks of burning light can be viewed from great distances. Sky's light shines like that, vast and bright and for all to see. Well when little Sky Burke came in to our offices and shared her story of advocacy and self-determination, my eyes began to flood with pride for her. One so small who had already learned by age 11 that our diversity is what makes us so special.

Sky's journey and the journey of the "Shining Stars" before her is the power of the journey of self. The voices of those heard and unheard. The voice of self -belief that can transcend all things, all titles, all diagnosis and create a world where all people can be all things. This is the place where Sky lives; this is the place where the Sky is limitless. Her story is the story of self-advocacy years in the making. The story and the testimony of civil rights activists speaking their truth for equal opportunity and freedom of choice. A movement started so long ago, and yet still underway.

Sky is part of that movement now. A leader in her own right who can support others for generations to come to believe in who they are. To choose who they wish to be. Statistics show that over 54 million Americans are people with disabilities. What statistics don't show are the successes, accomplishments and drive of these individuals. Over the past 3 and half years I have spent at the Self-Advocacy Association of NYS I have encountered more talented, compassionate and accepting individuals than I have in almost all of my 40 years. Their spirits, innovations and determination are unrivaled. This time has been one of the greatest learning experiences of my life to date.

To look inside ourselves and find that place where all things are possible. Where each person's talents and abilities are acknowledged and nurtured is the greatest gift we can give to ourselves and those around us. In supporting one another we support ourselves and our own abilities to reach higher and believe for more. More choices, more freedom, more humanity. And then, and only then can we live in the place where Sky does. The place where the SKY is limitless.

Written By, Bridget M. Cariello

I am many things.
I am a girl.
I am 10 years old and
I have a very cool name.
It's Sky.

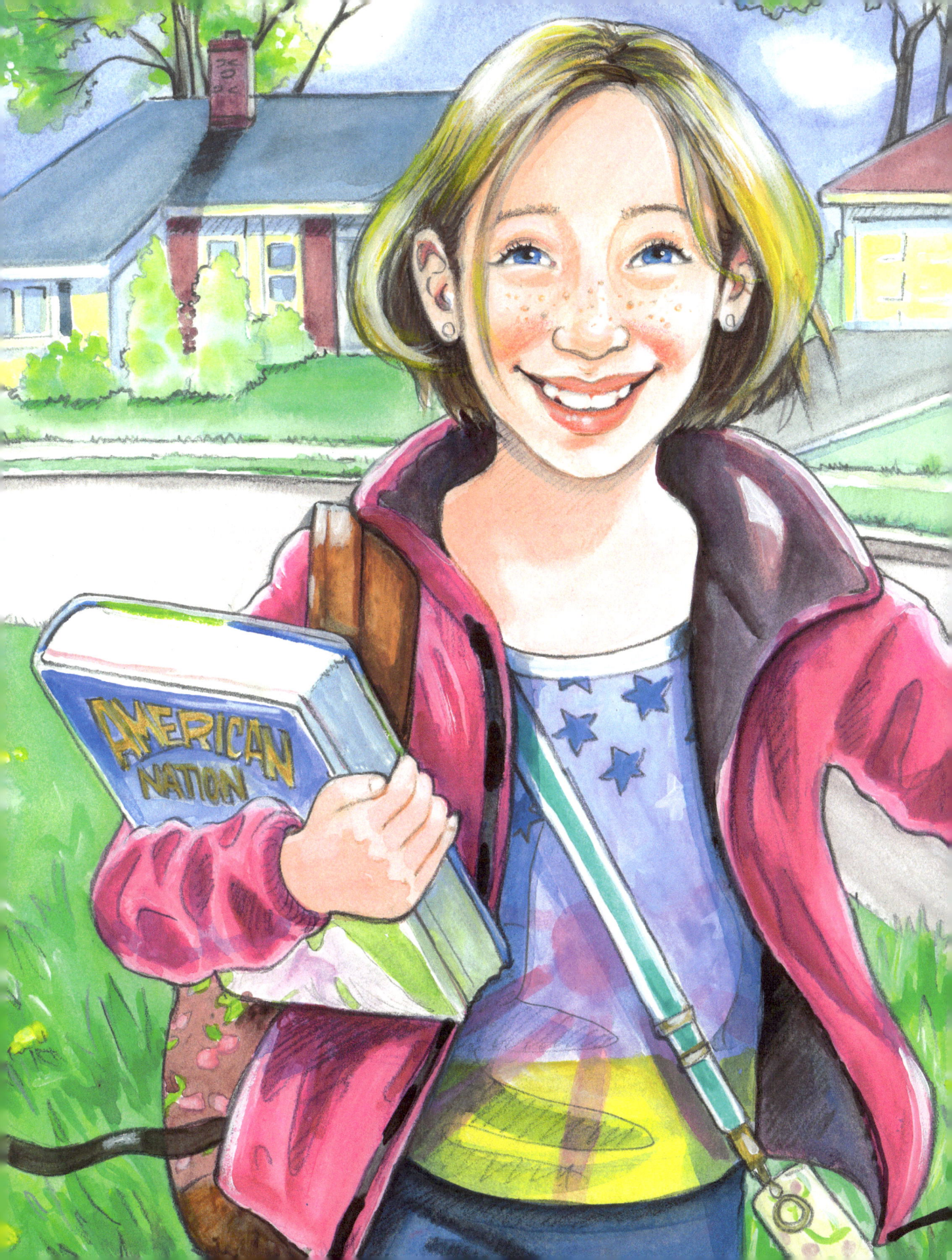

I am a good student, now. But I was not always.
I used to be nervous in school.

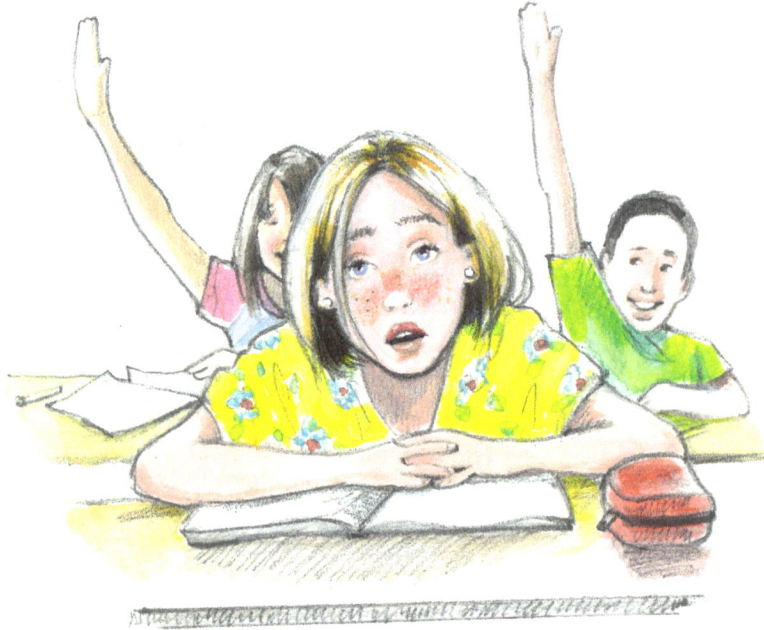

In third grade I couldn't read and I couldn't
write, at least, not very well.

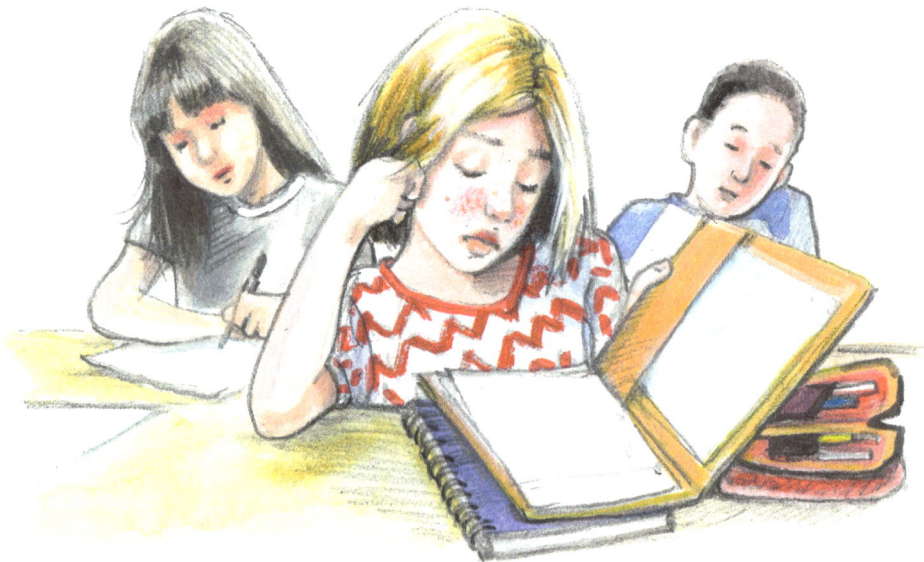

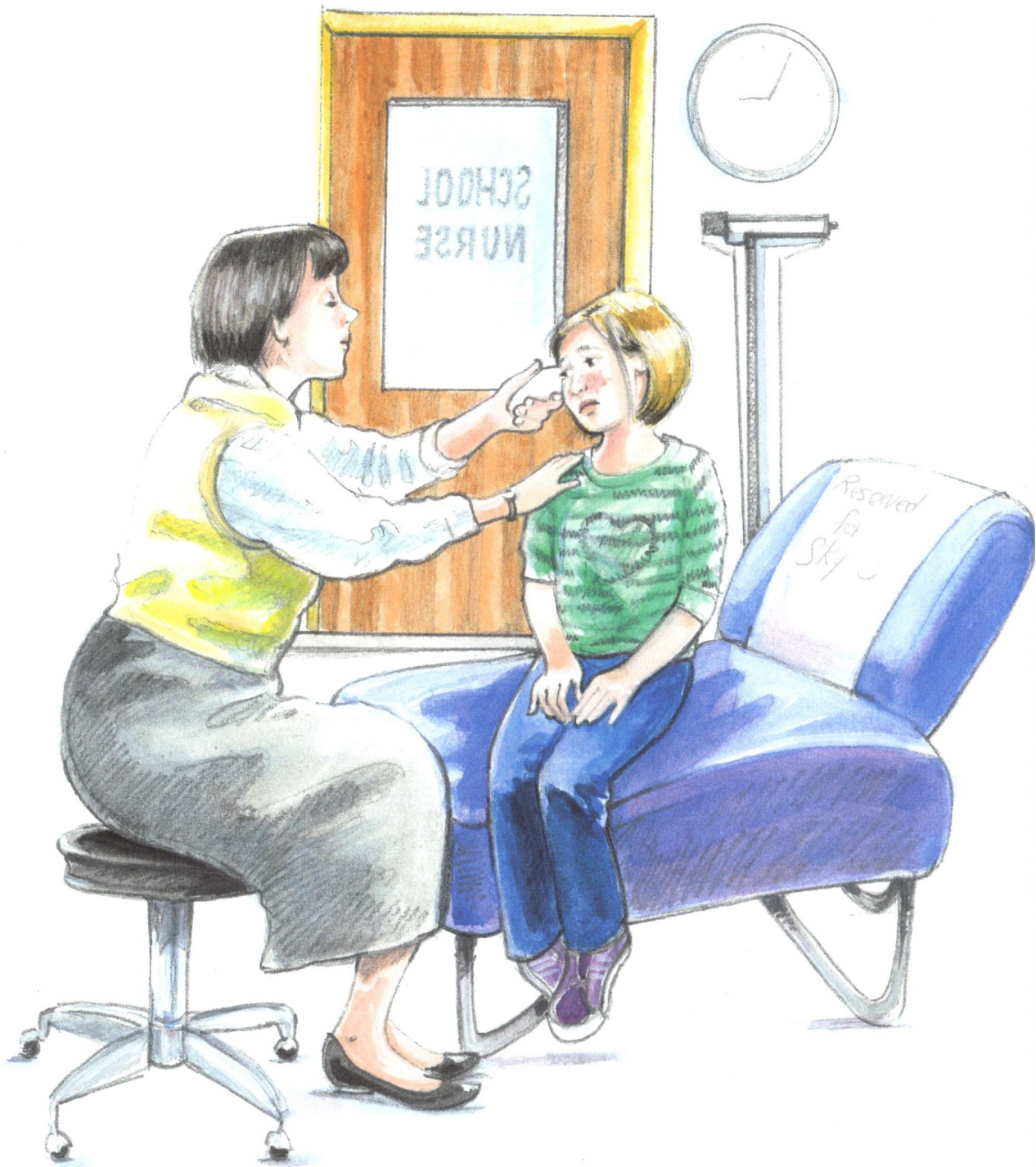

My head ached and I went to the nurse.
A lot.

Soon my mom took me to a doctor.

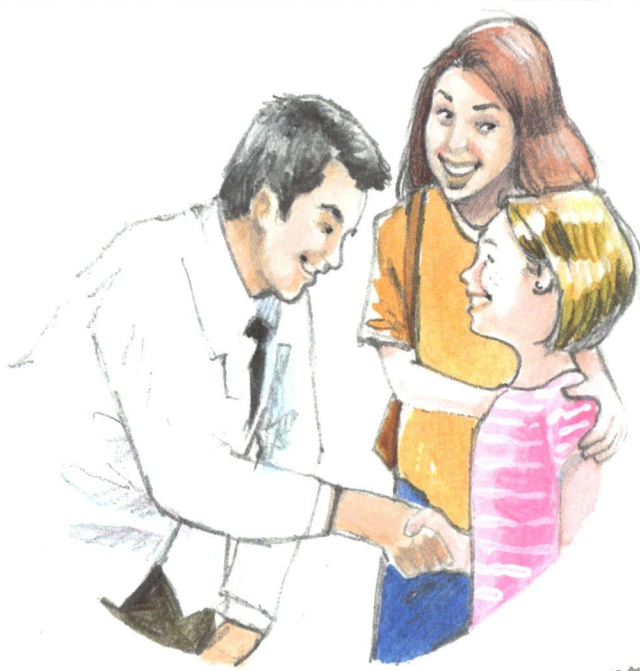

He asked me lots of questions.

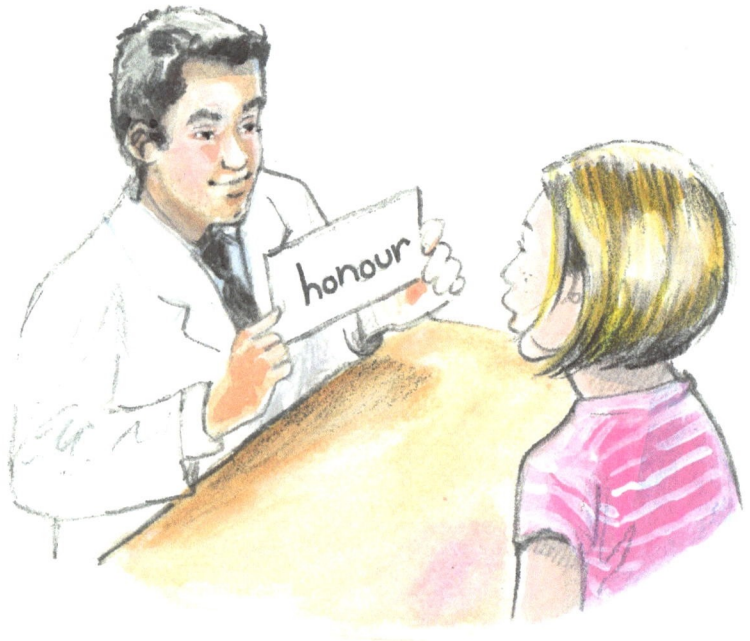

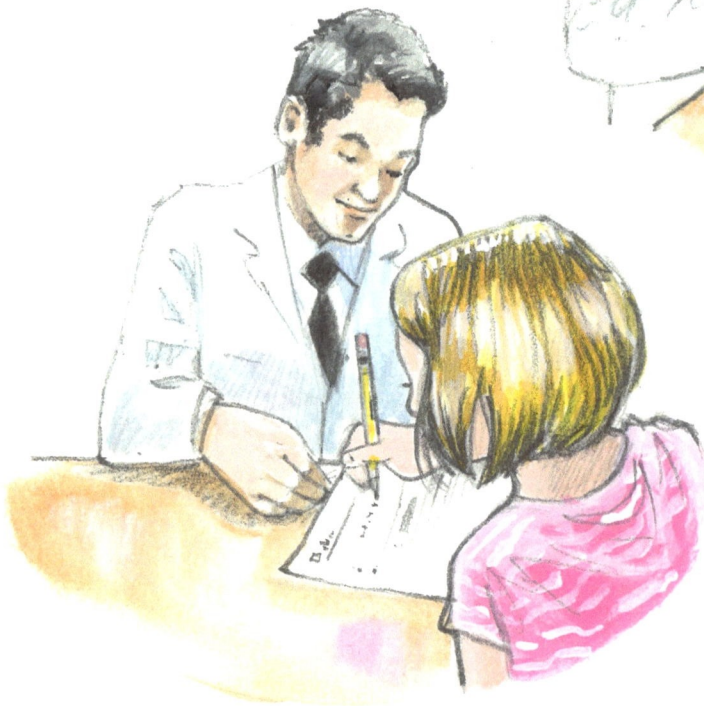

honour

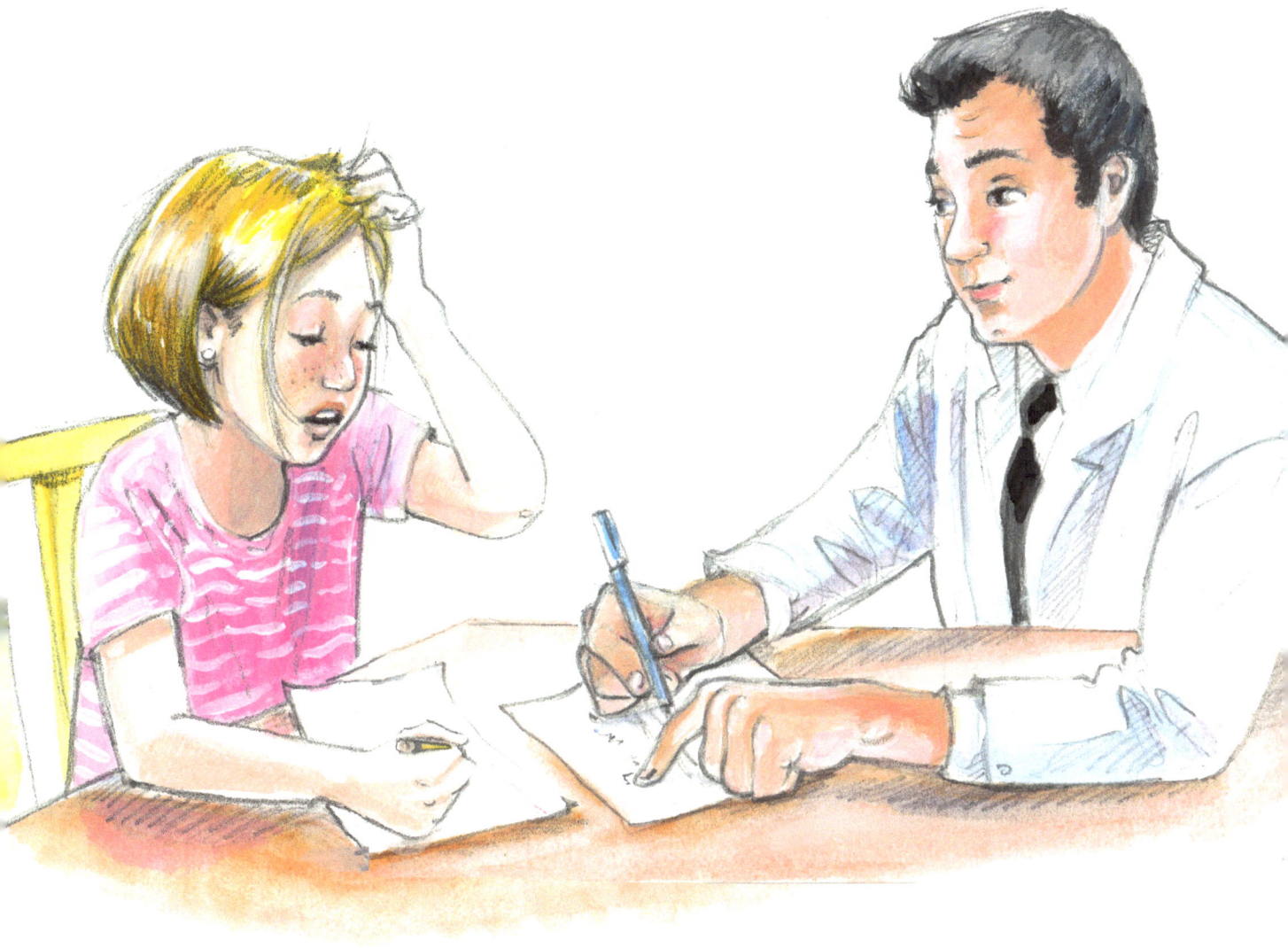

He gave me tests!

He told my mom many things and used big words
that I didn't understand.
I thought everyone had trouble
reading and writing.

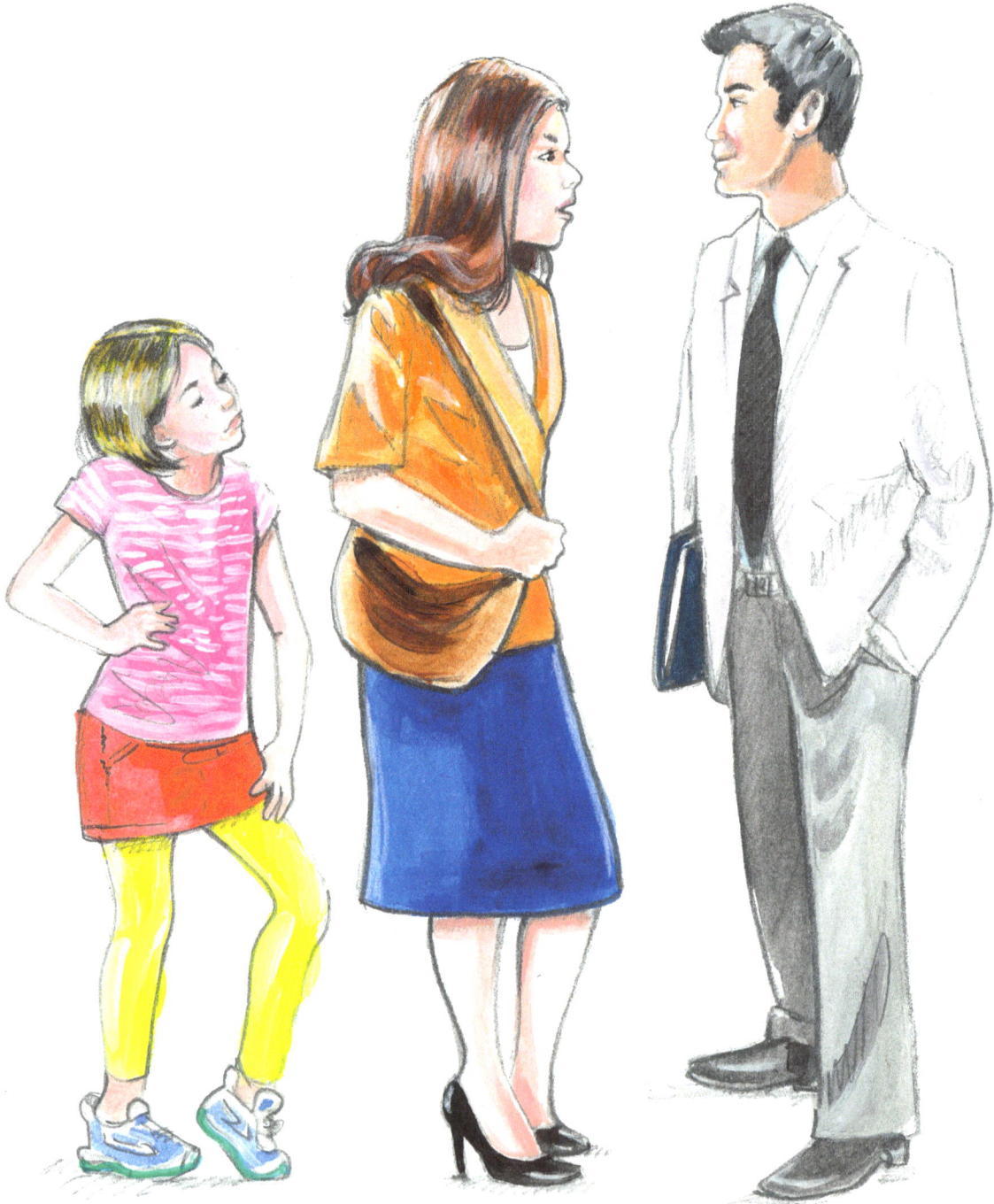

Readthisparagraph

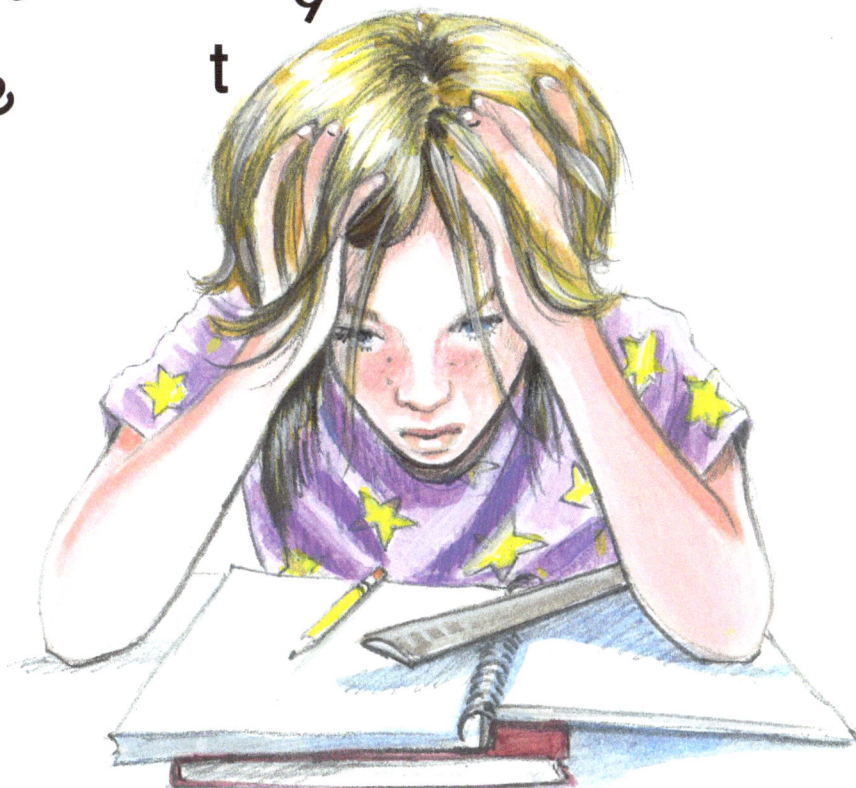

But now I am older.
The big words my doctor used were
Dyslexia and Dysgraphia.
When you have Dyslexia and Dysgraphia
words and letters jump around before your eyes.
That's what was happening to me!

My mom and I went to a lot of meetings and I listened to grownups talk, and talk and talk. My mom said that a 8 year old kid was not expected to attend.

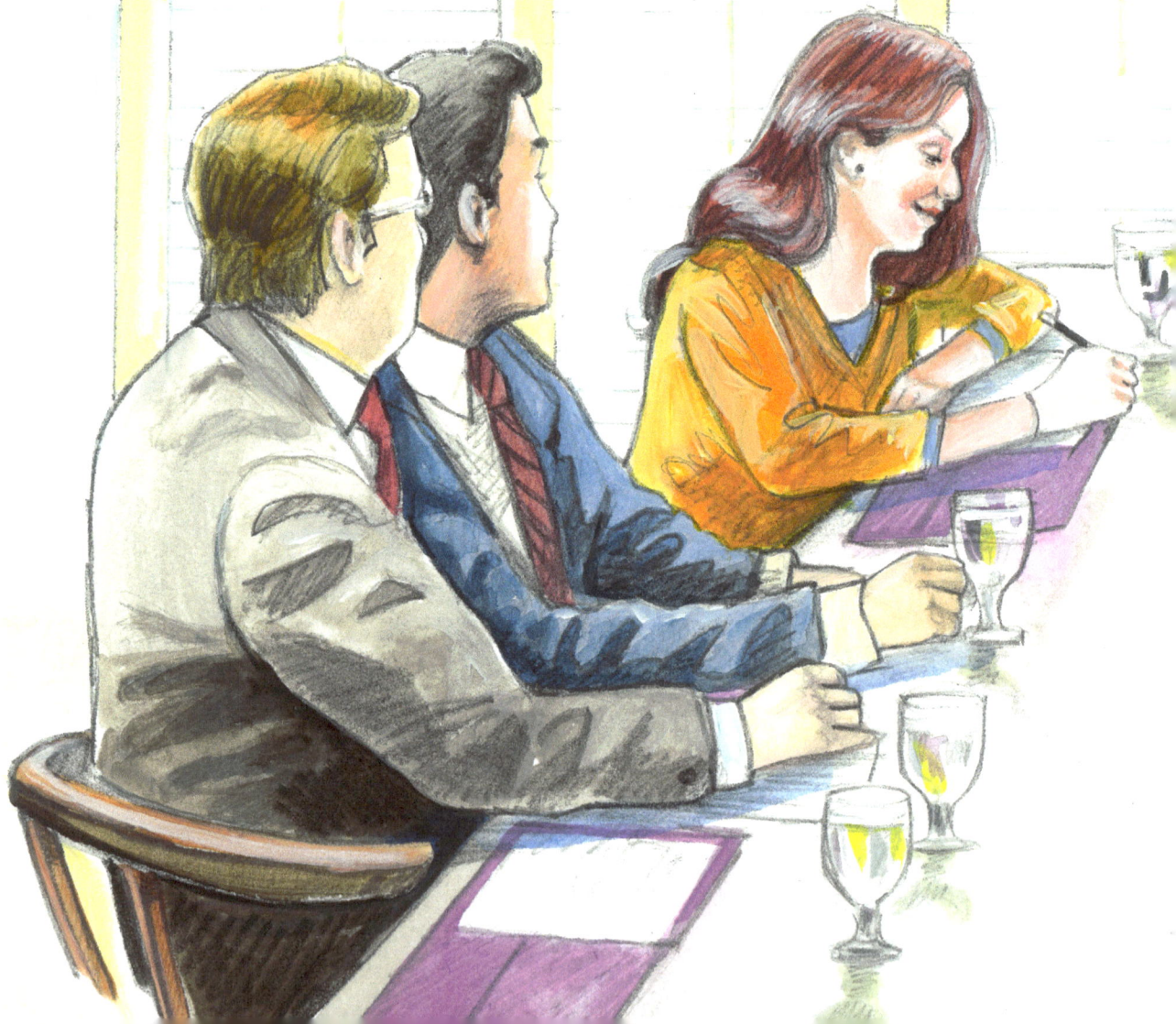

But I thought I should. After all, they were all talking about me!

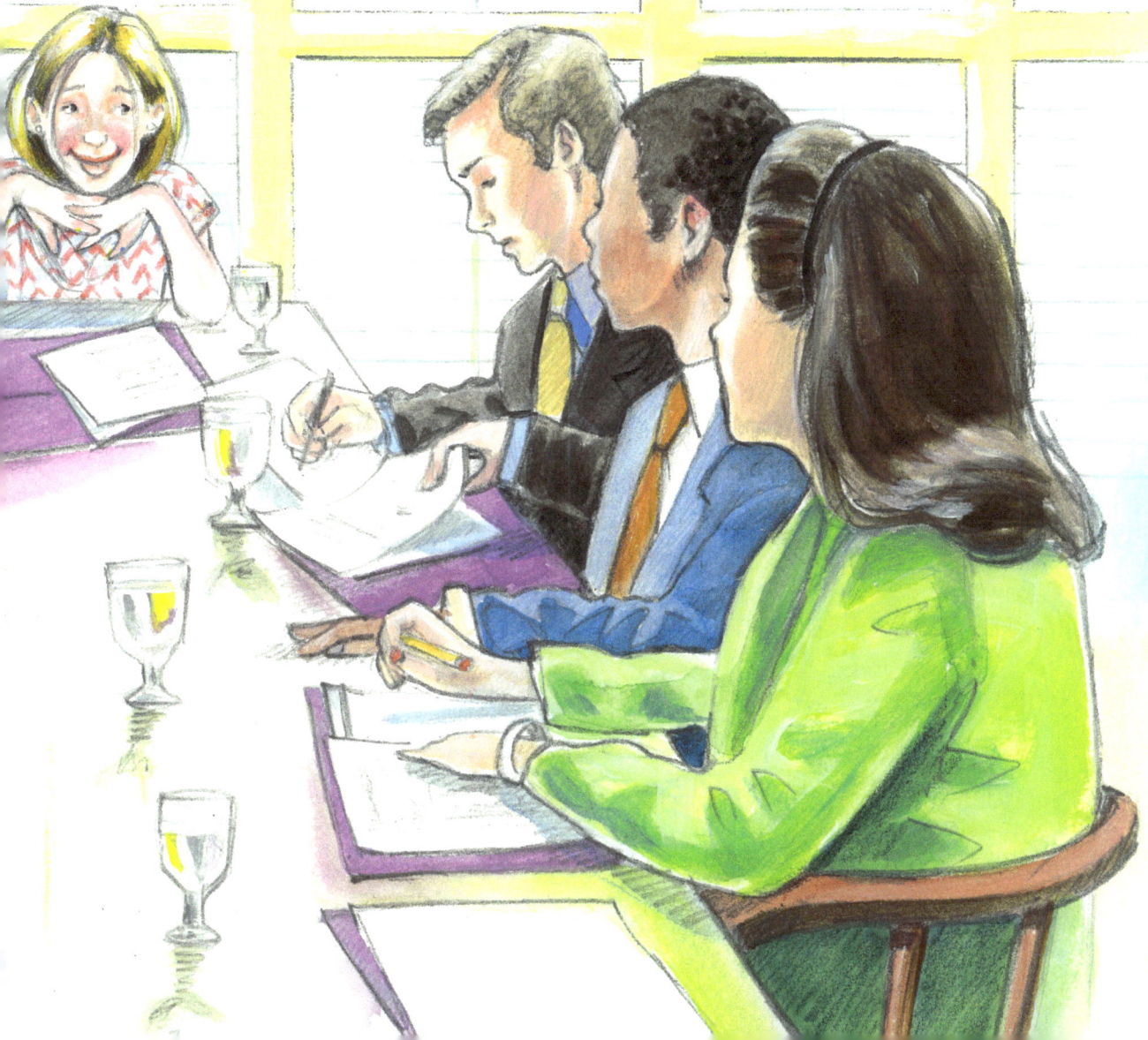

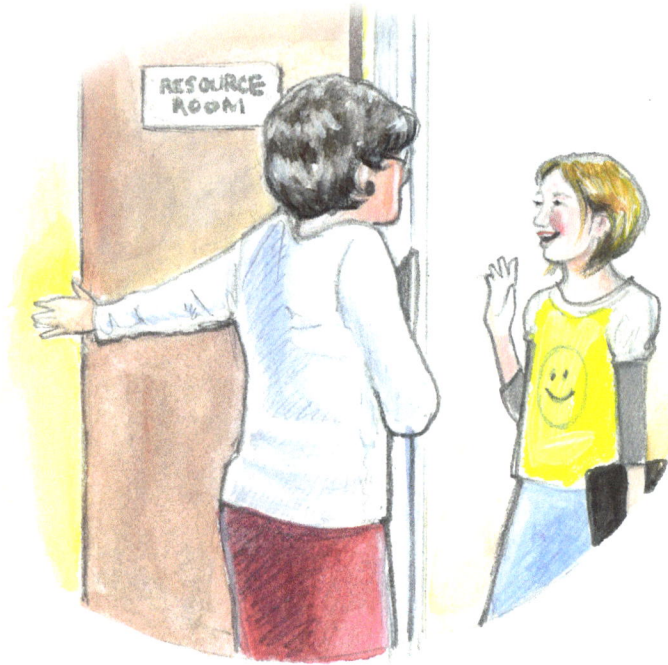

I began visiting new teachers during school.
I was given extra time on tests.

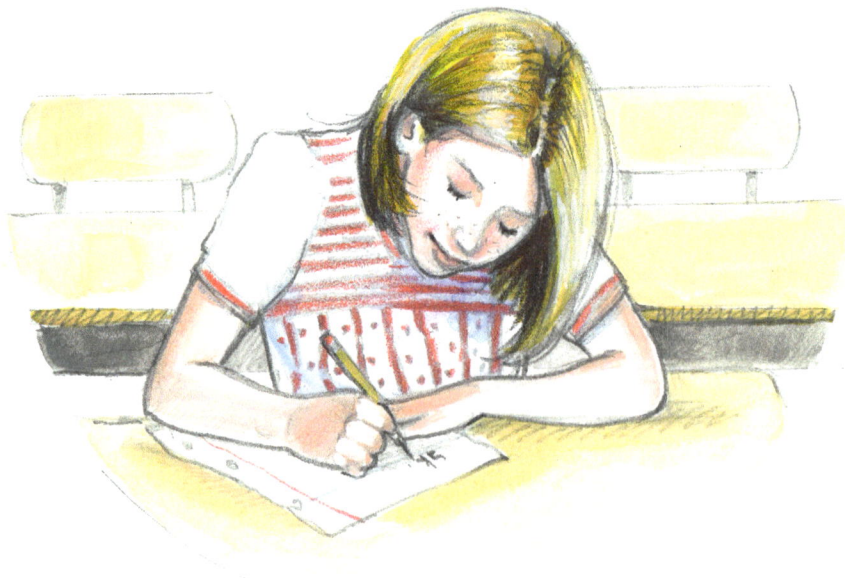

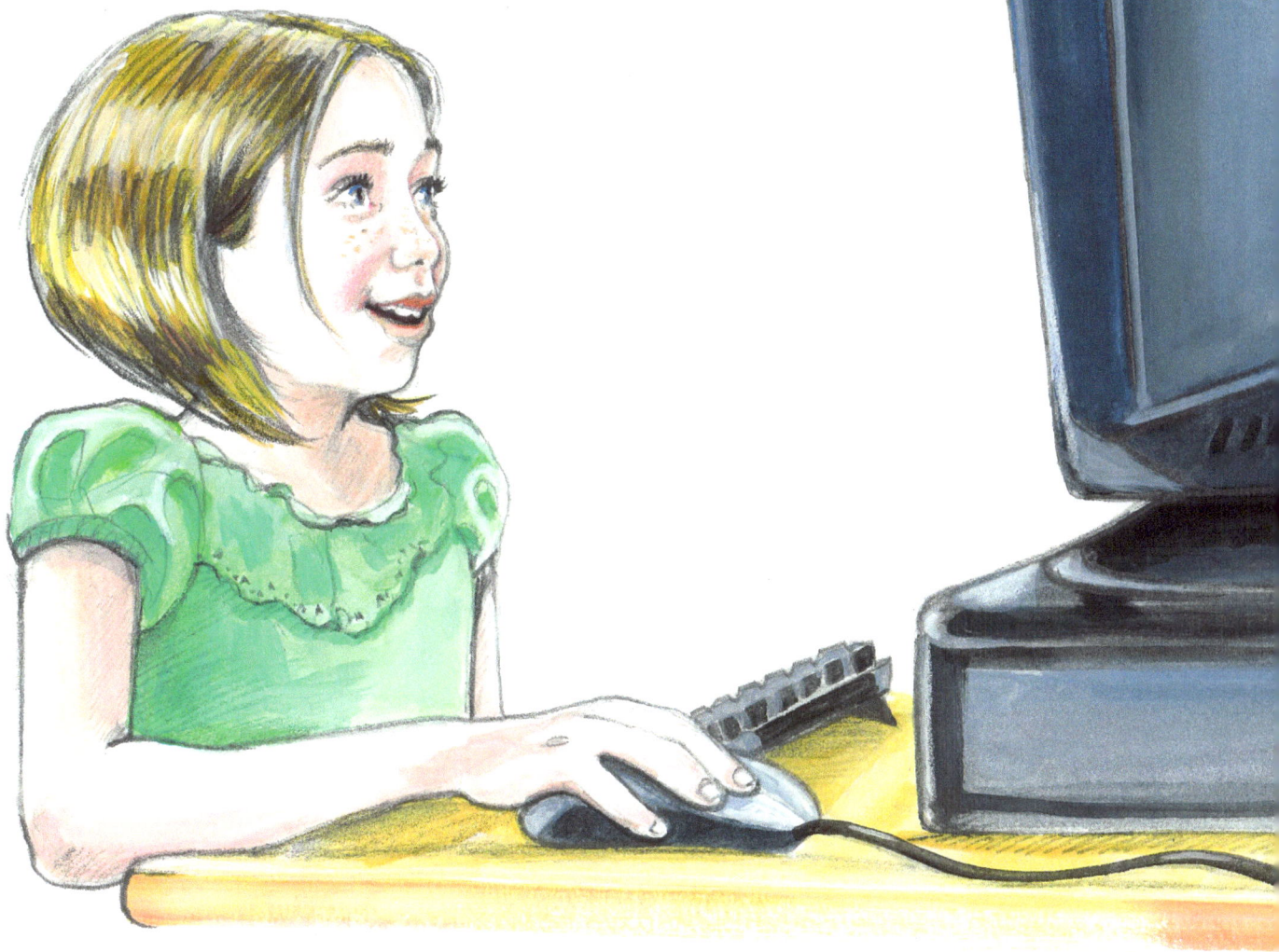

I even got to play on special computers.

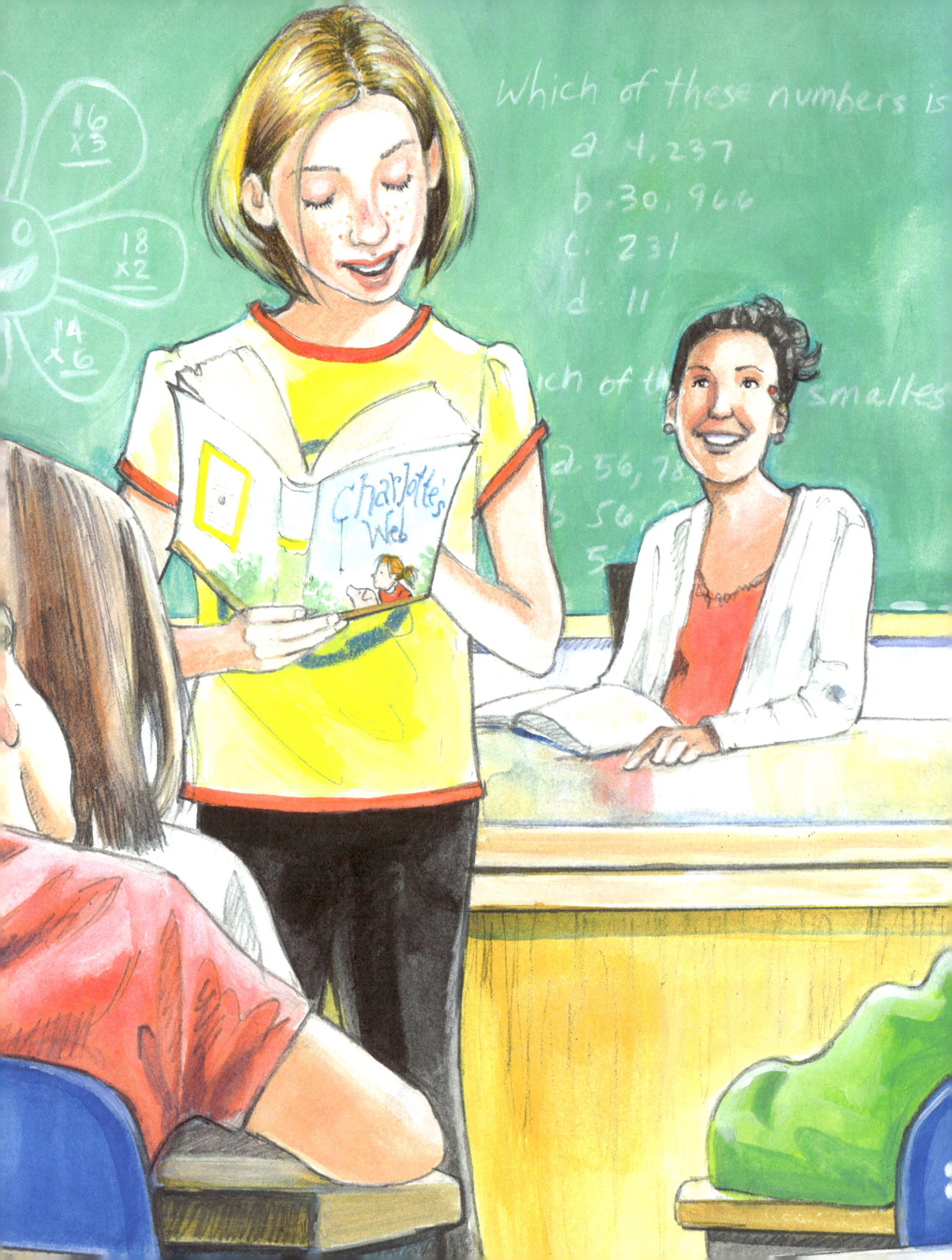

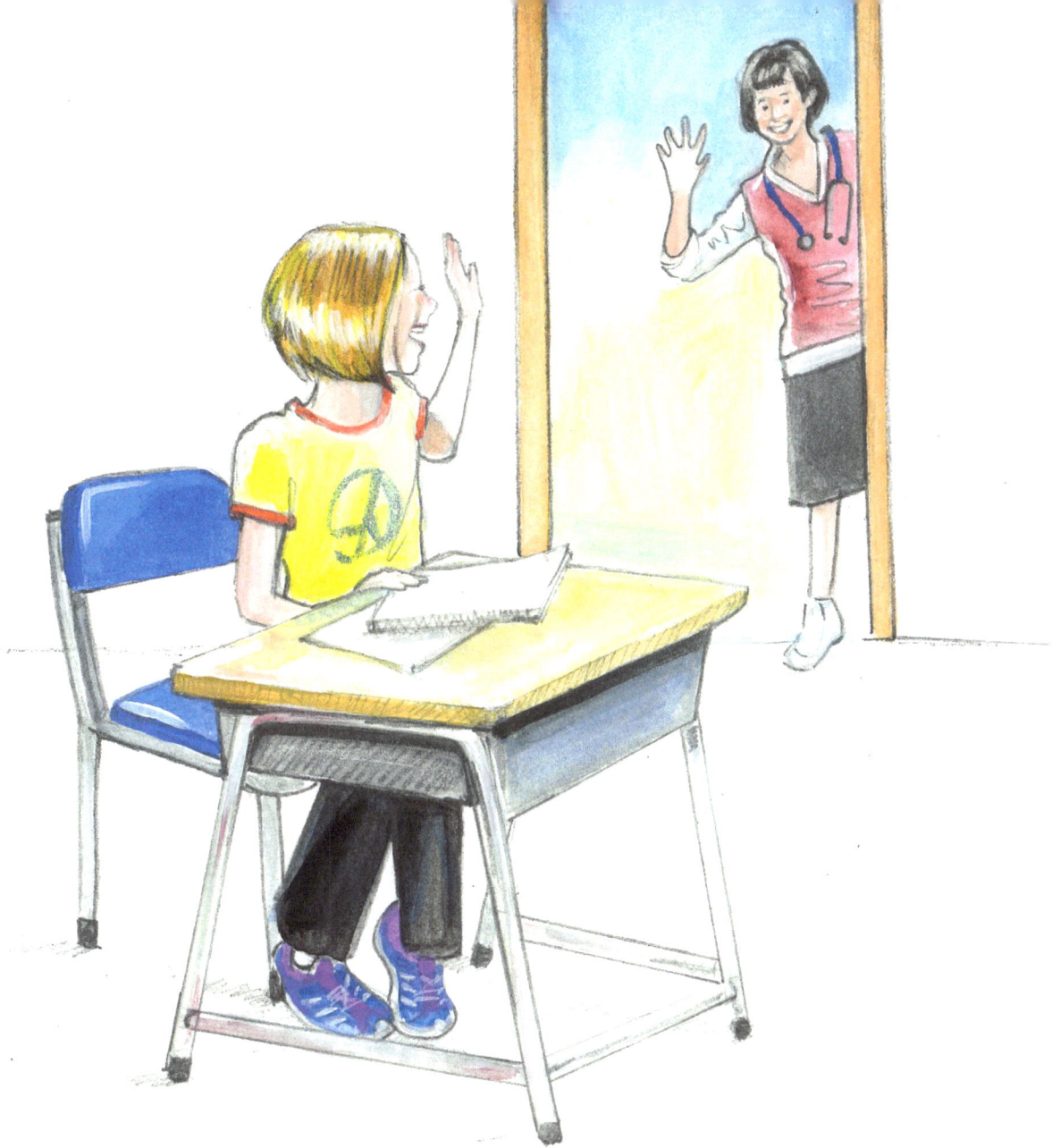

Soon I could read and write much better!
And the nurse had to come
to visit me to say hello.

But I still wanted to be
a better student.
Most of the other kids
worked fast.

I was slow.

Then my mom gave me
an iPad.

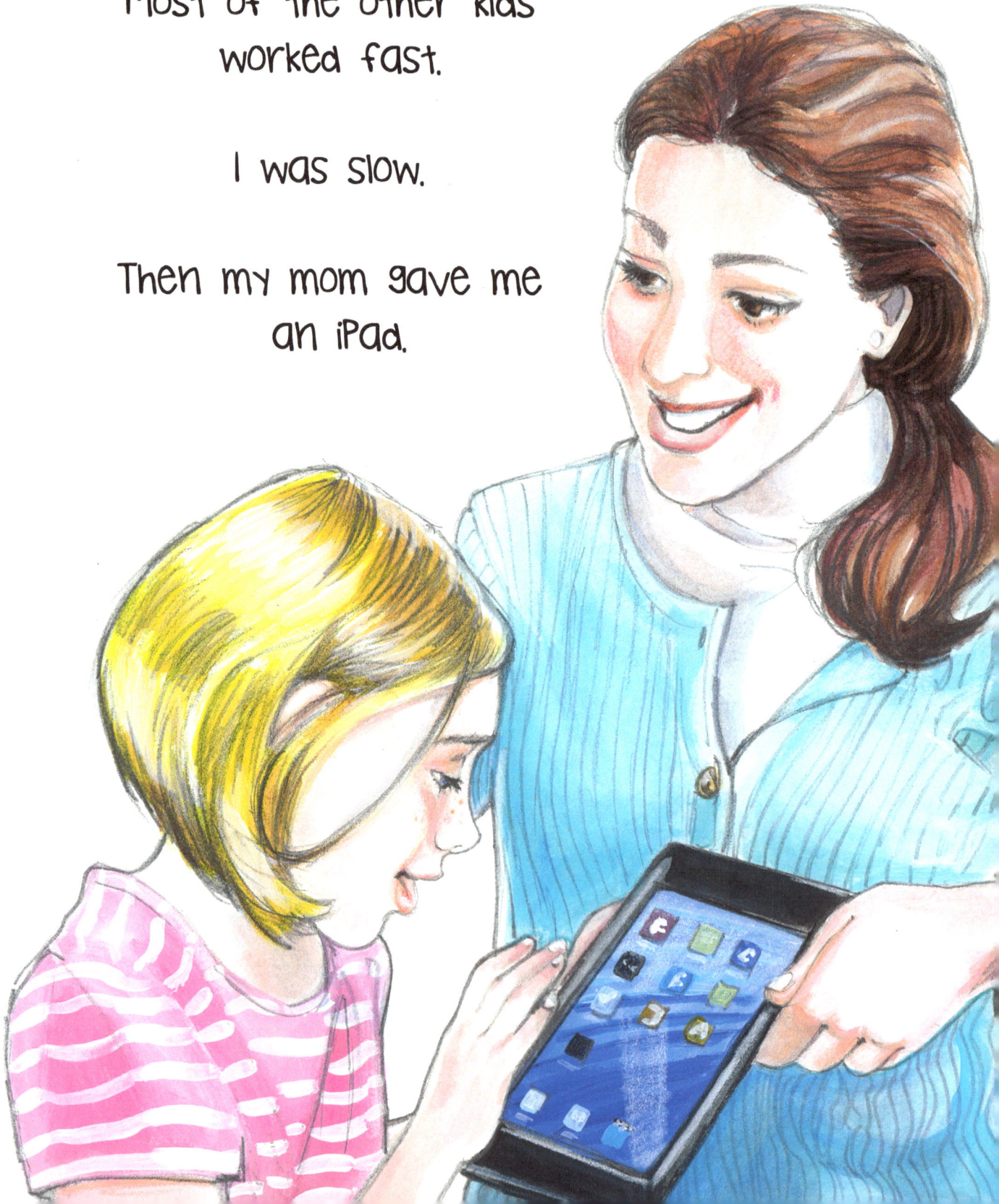

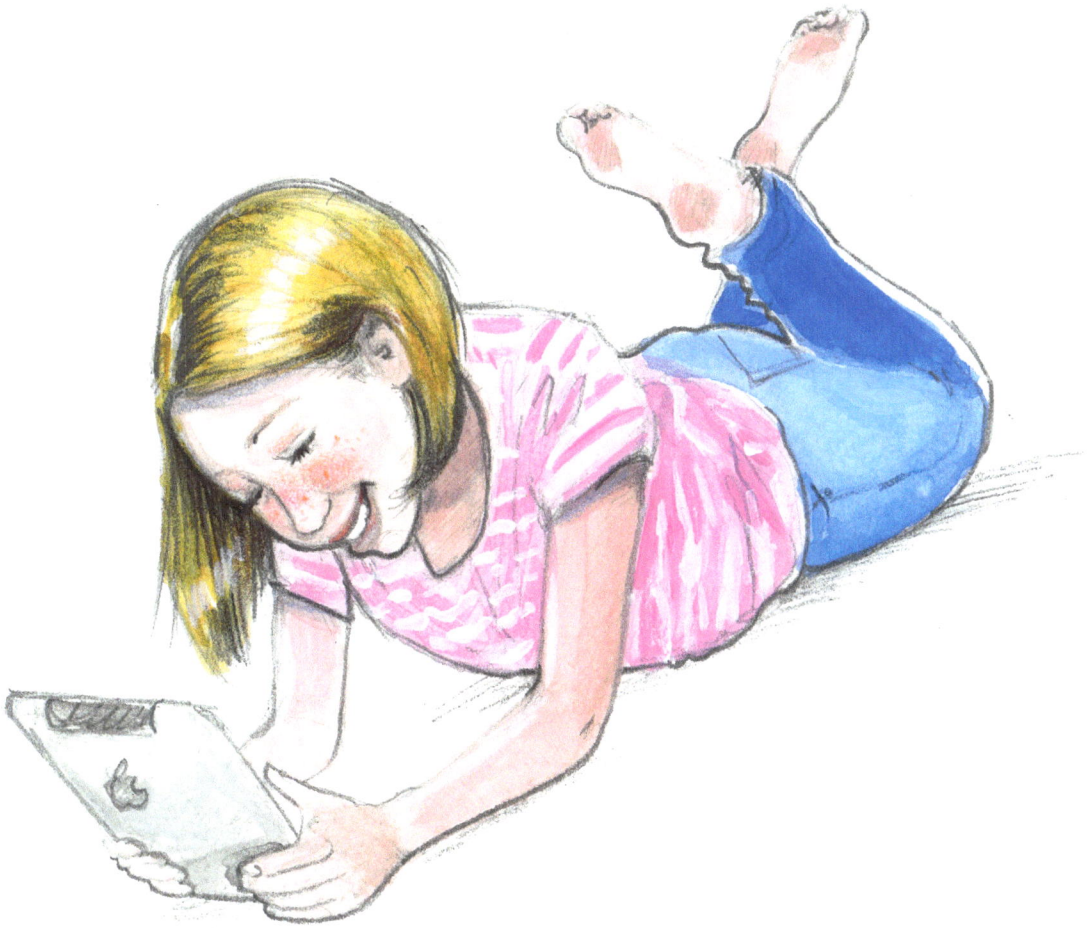

It was my most favorite gift ever!
My iPad helped me so much that,

after more meetings and more talking

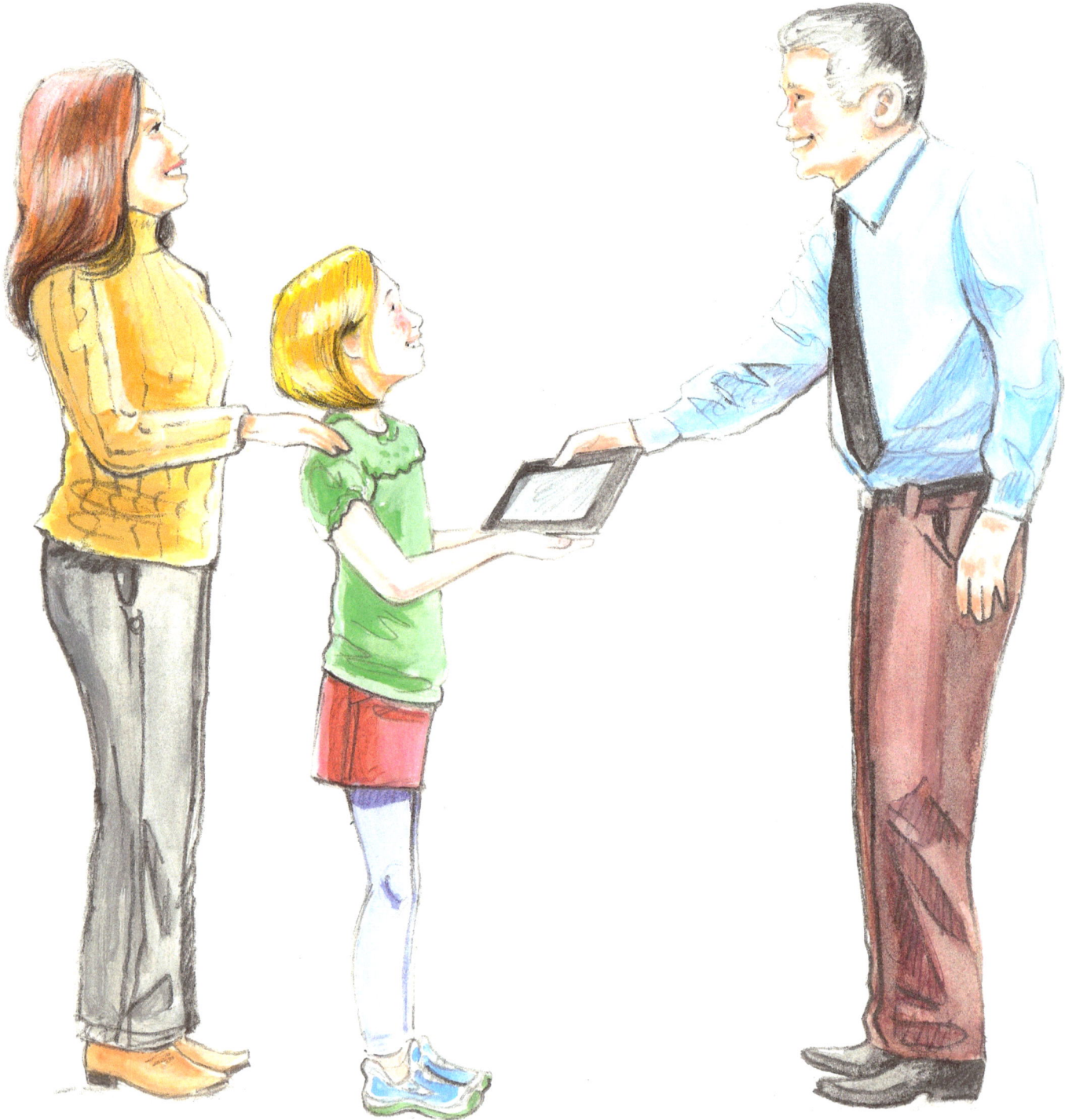

the teachers, the nurse, the principal and even the superintendent of schools decided to let me use my iPad in school.

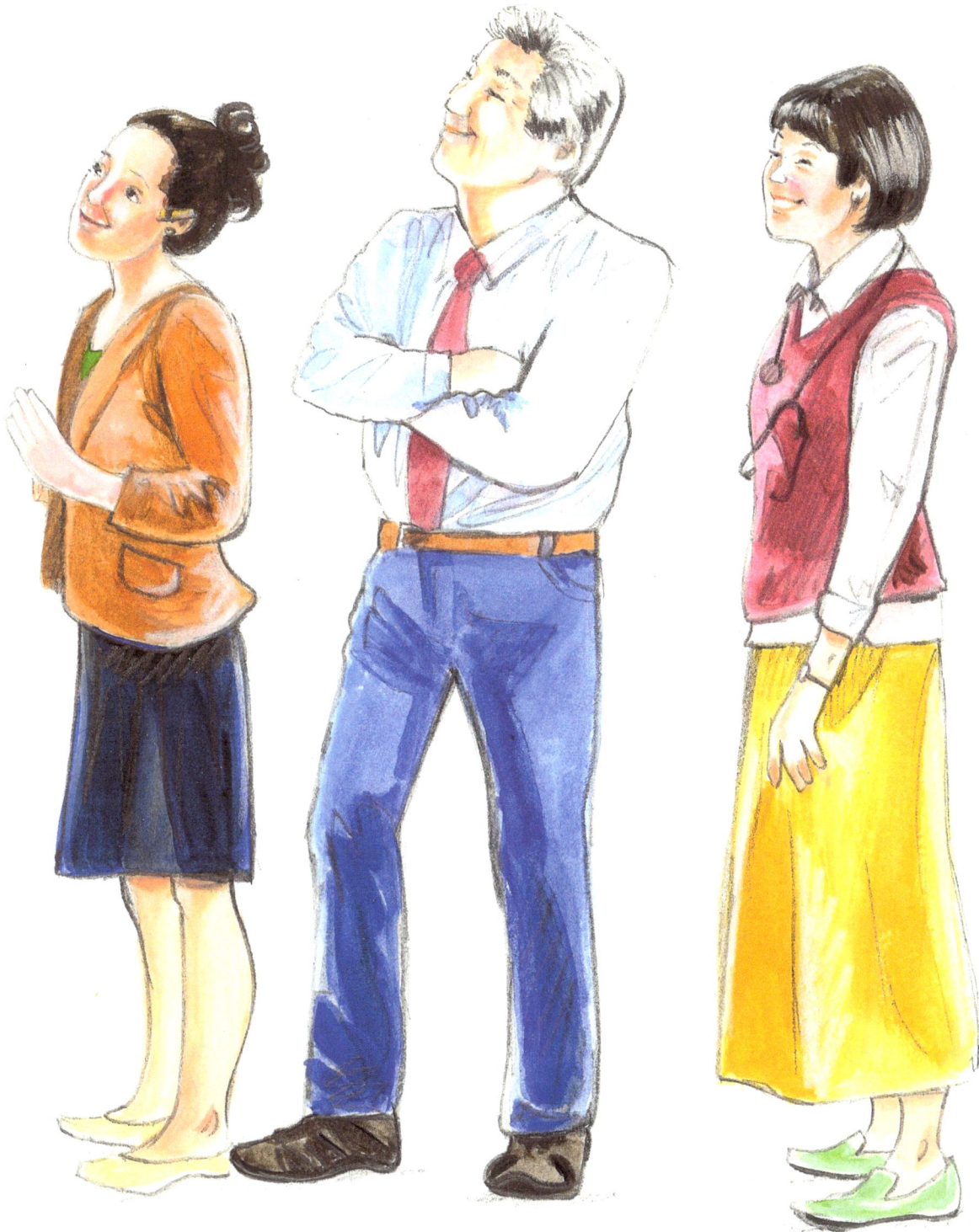

Now I tell everyone about how my iPad helps me.

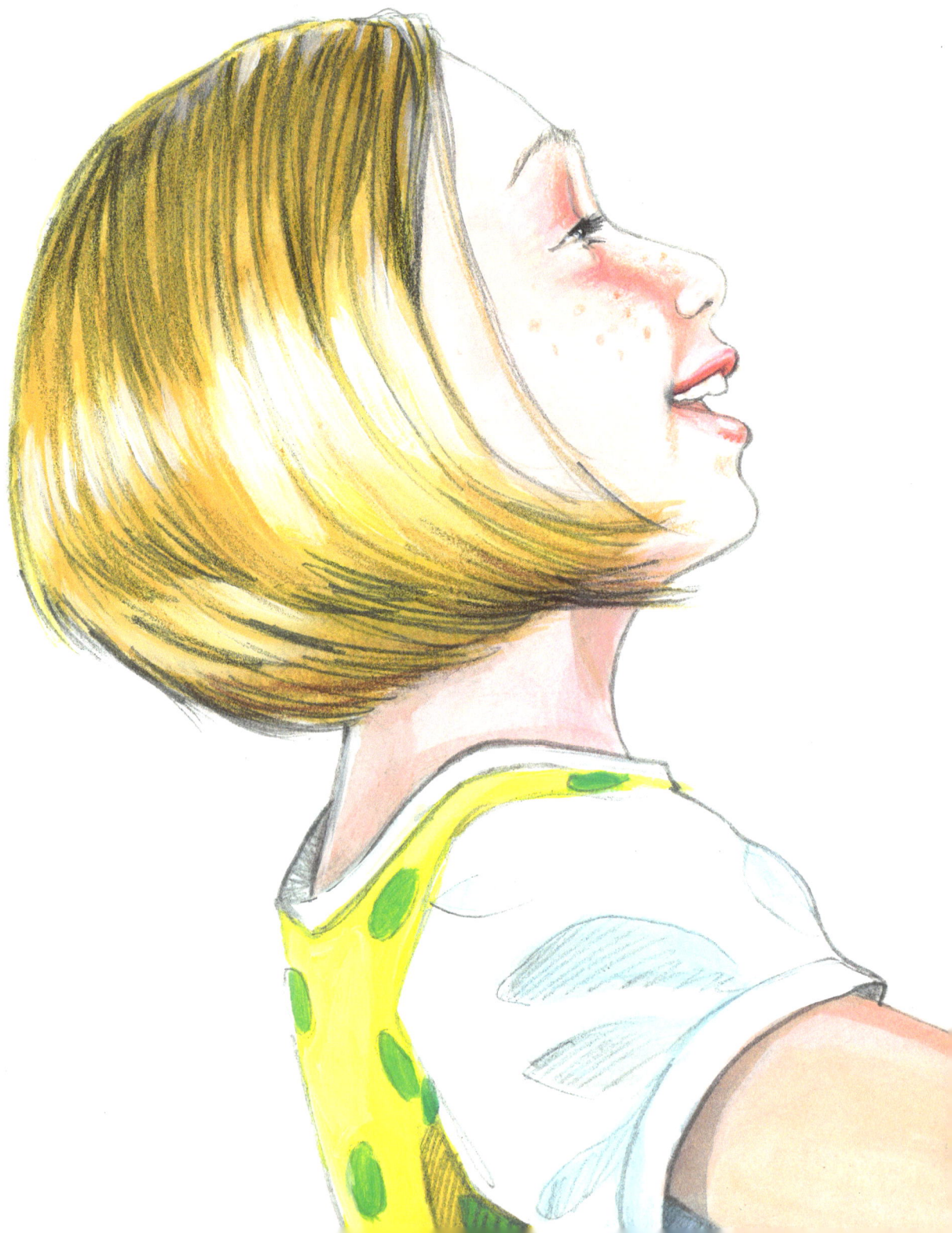

I talk to crowds of people into a loud microphone so everyone can hear me.

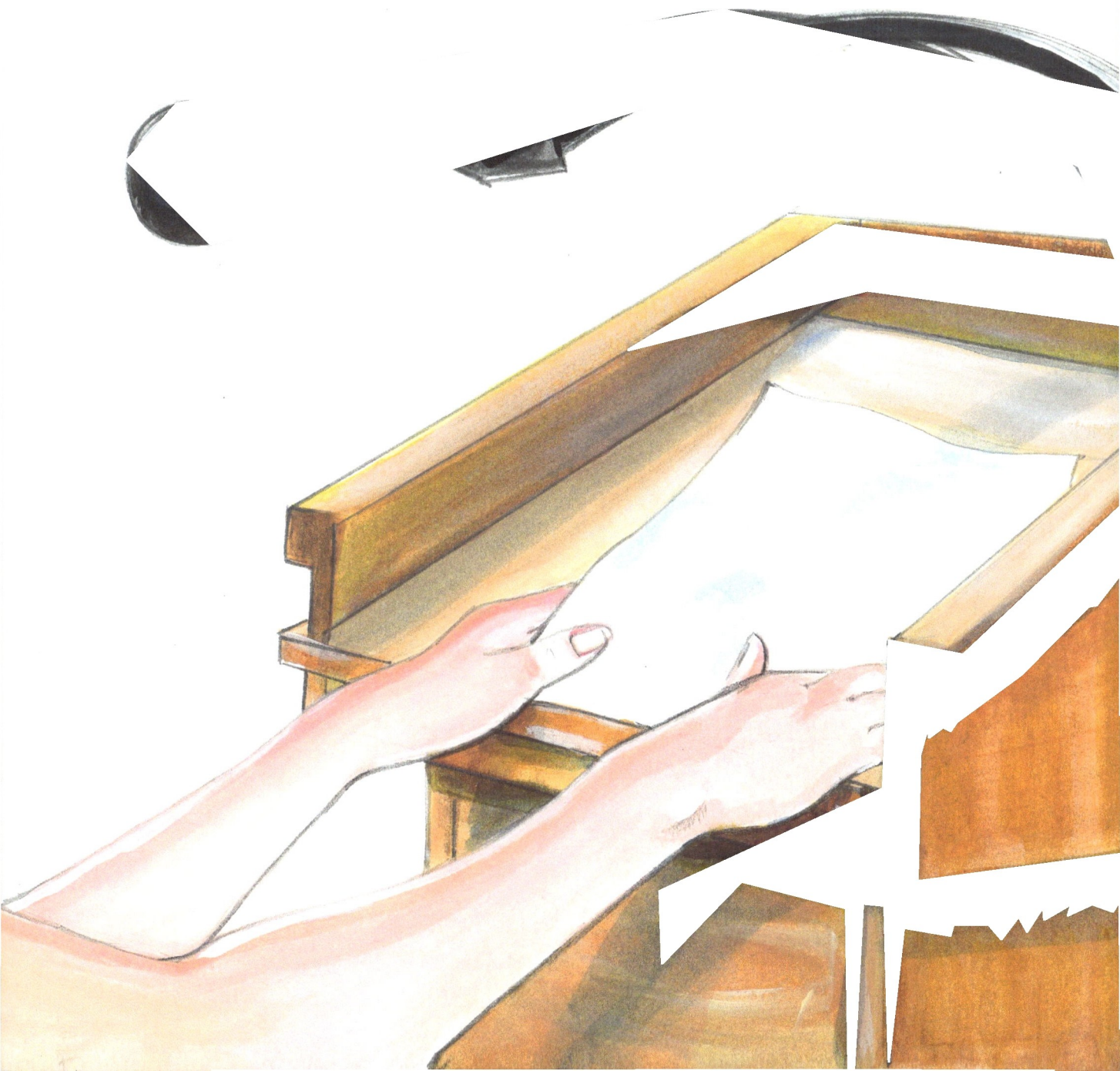

I say,
"I am Sky.
I have Dyslexia and Dysgraphia.
But that is not who I am."

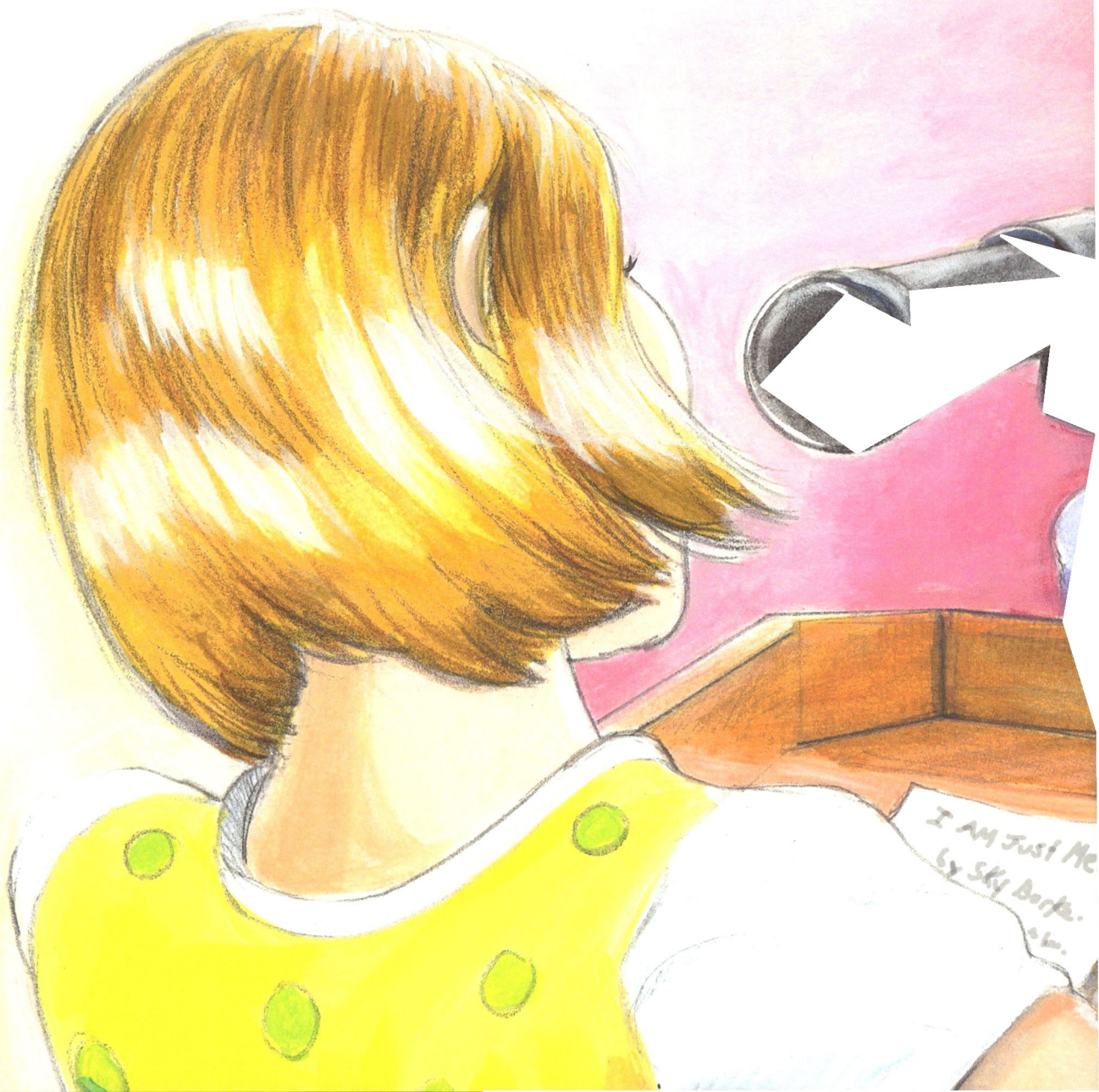

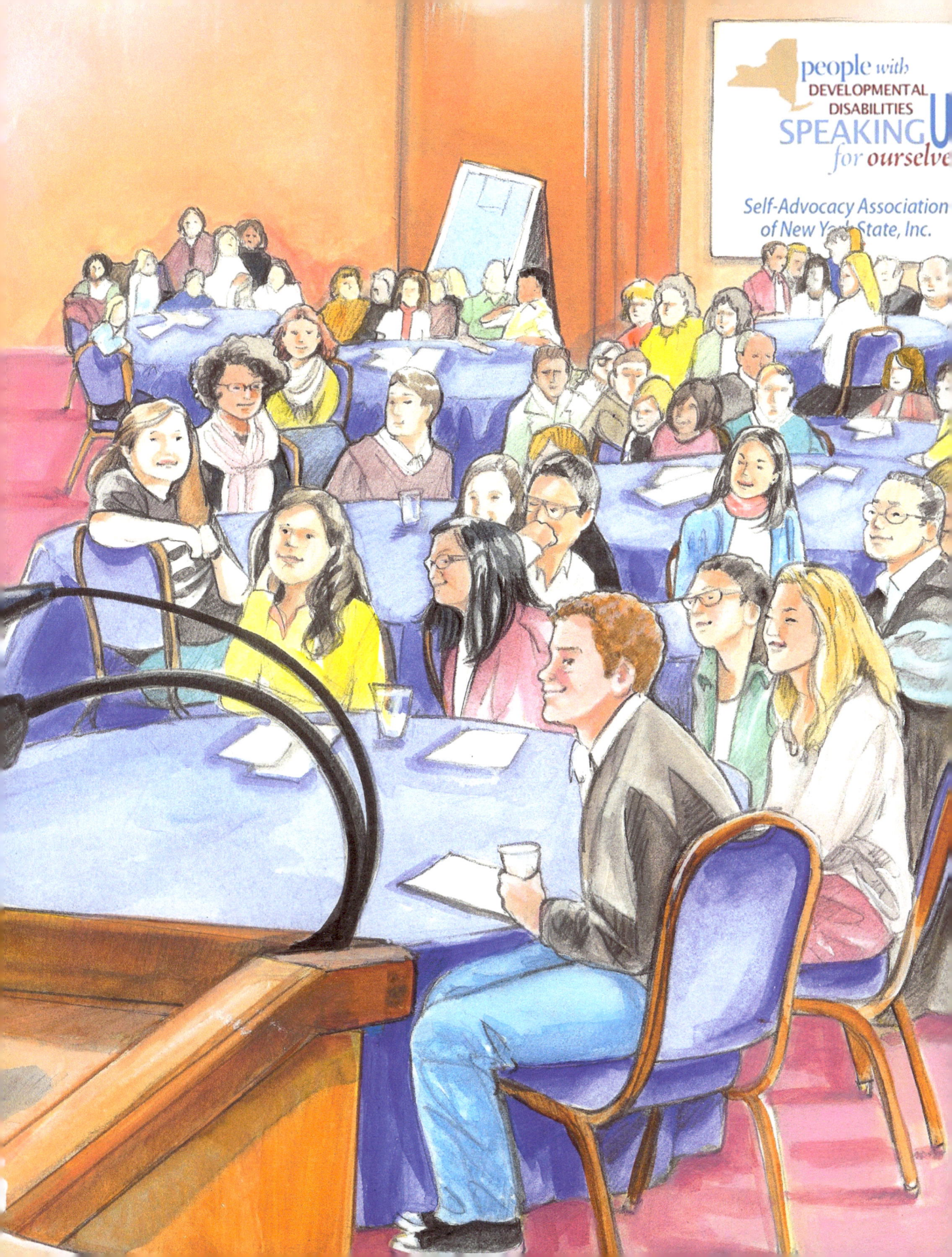

people with
DEVELOPMENTAL
DISABILITIES
SPEAKING UP
for ourselves

Self-Advocacy Association
of New York State, Inc.

"I am a flute player.

I am a singer.

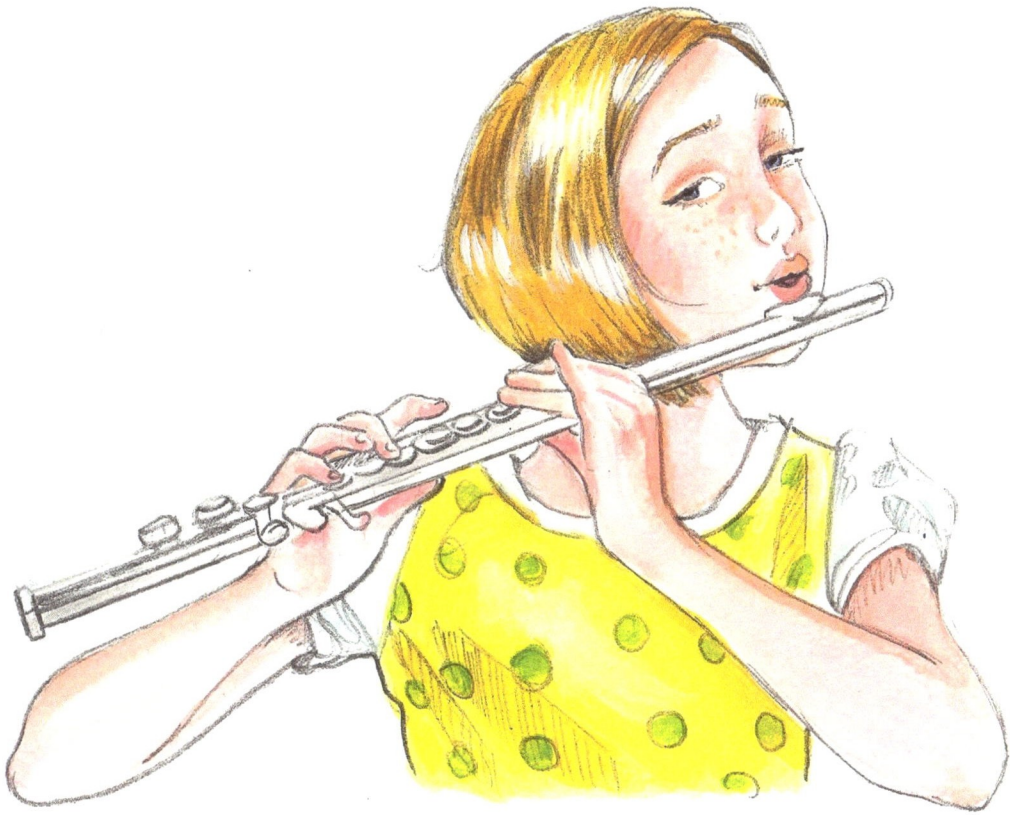

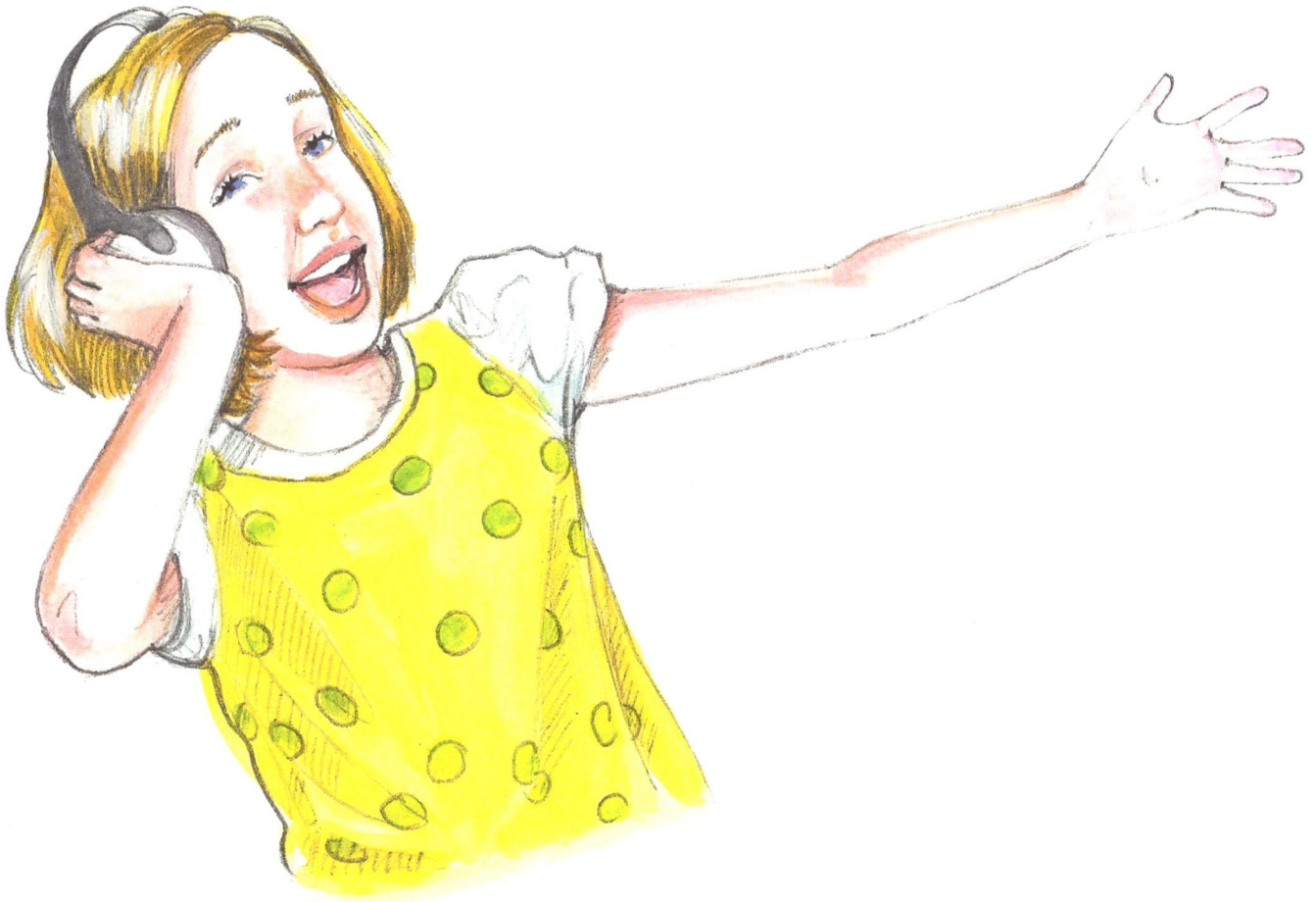

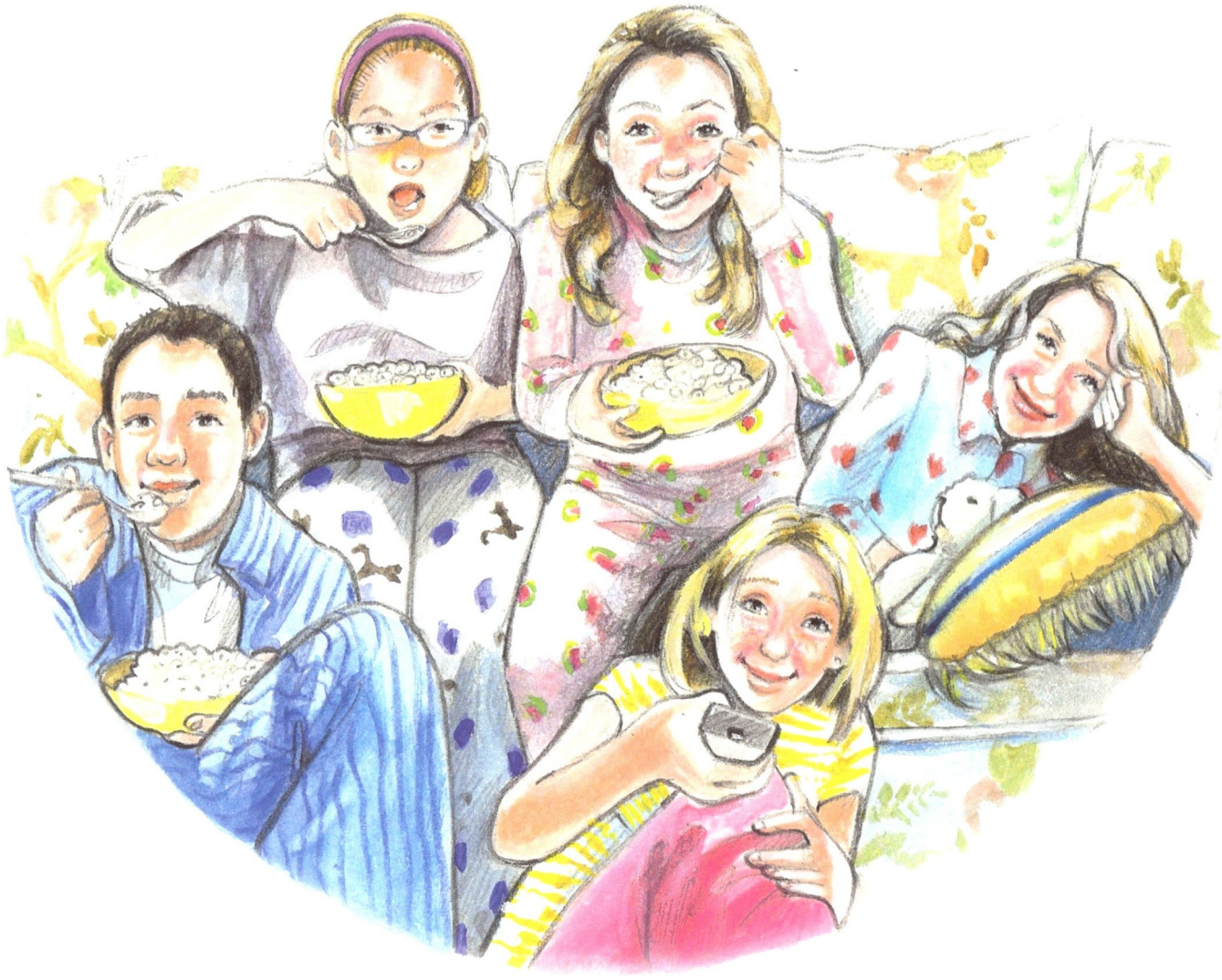

I am a good sister

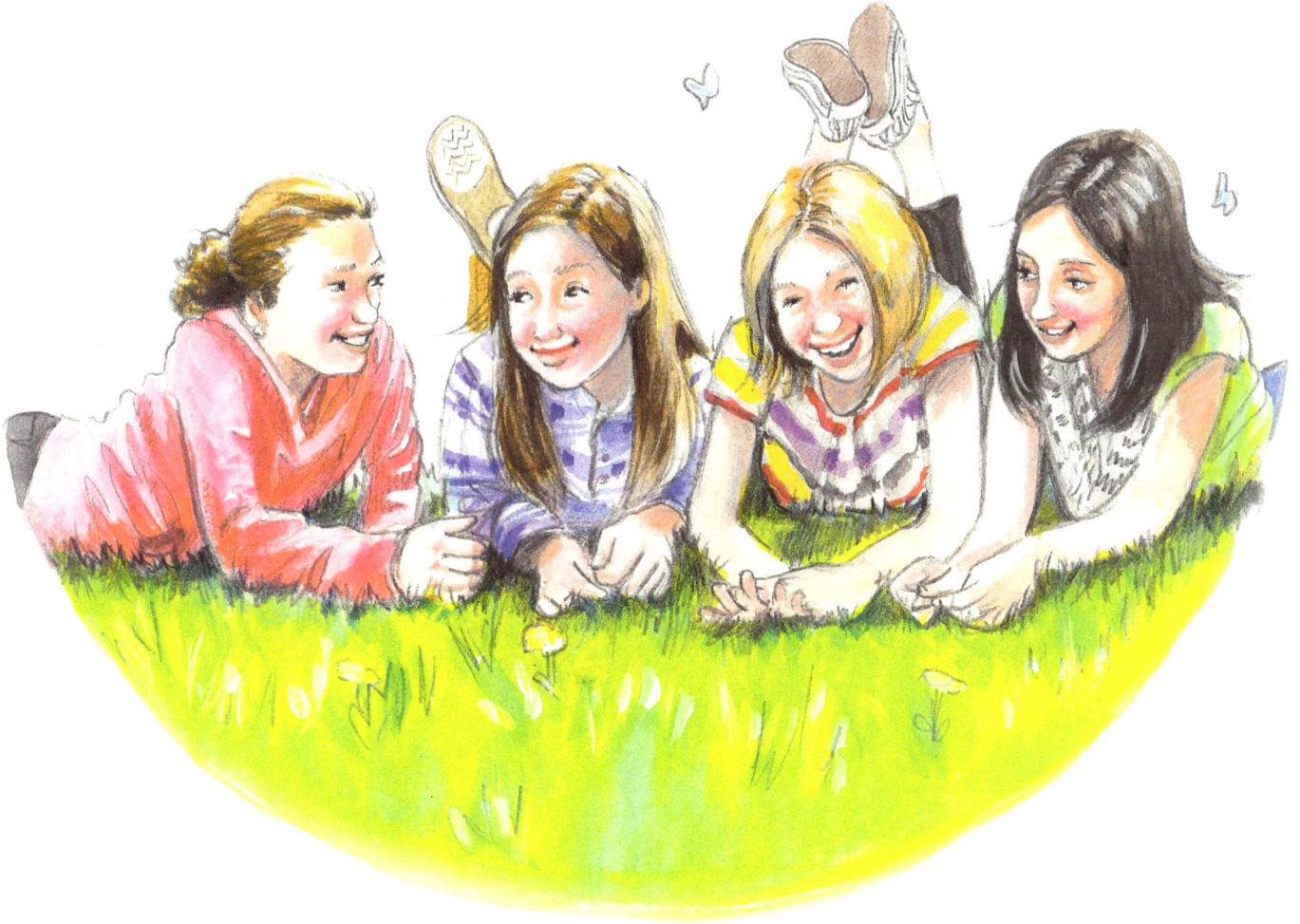

and a good friend.

I am a self-advocate."

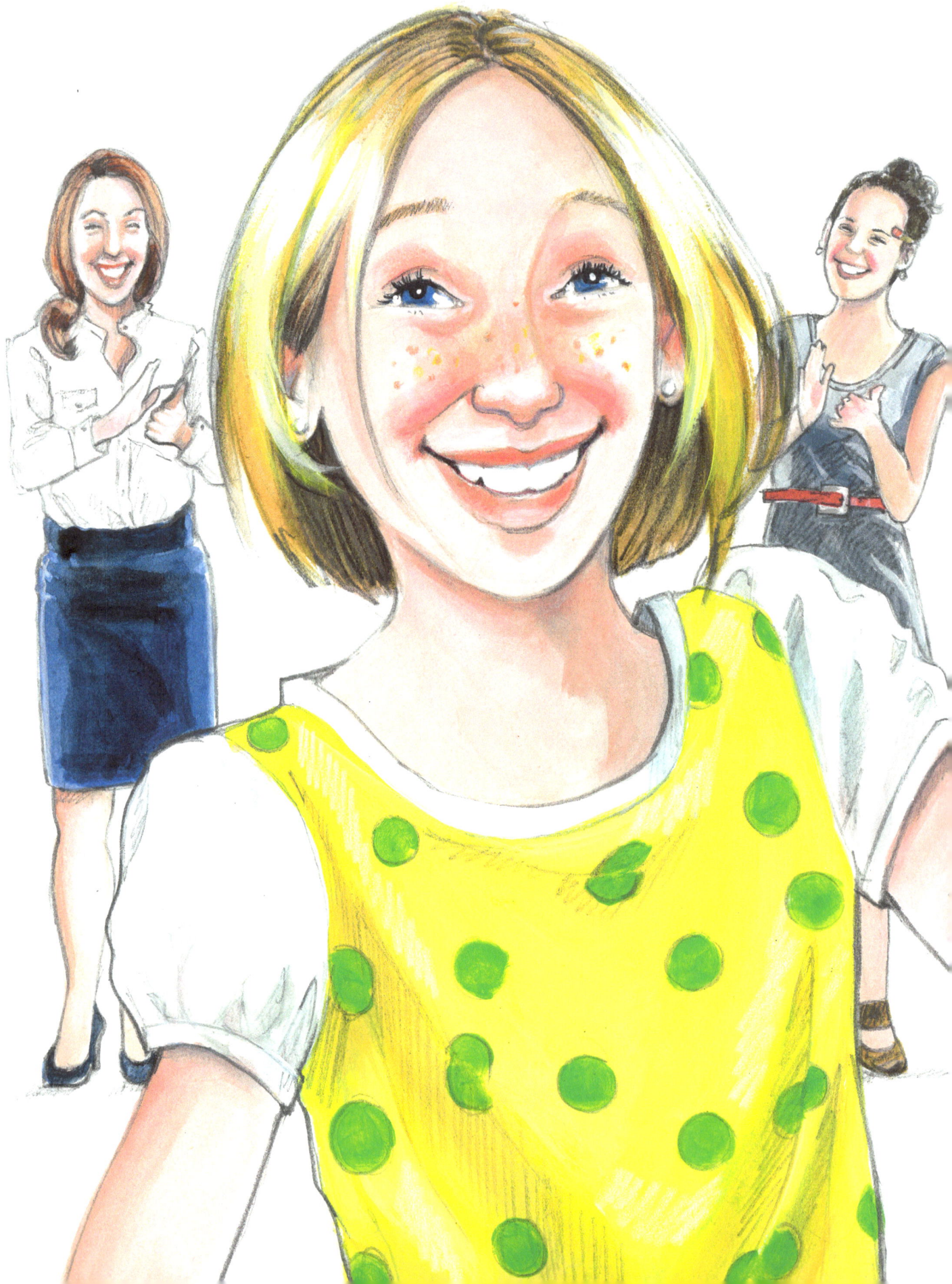

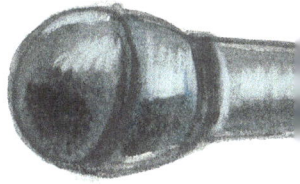
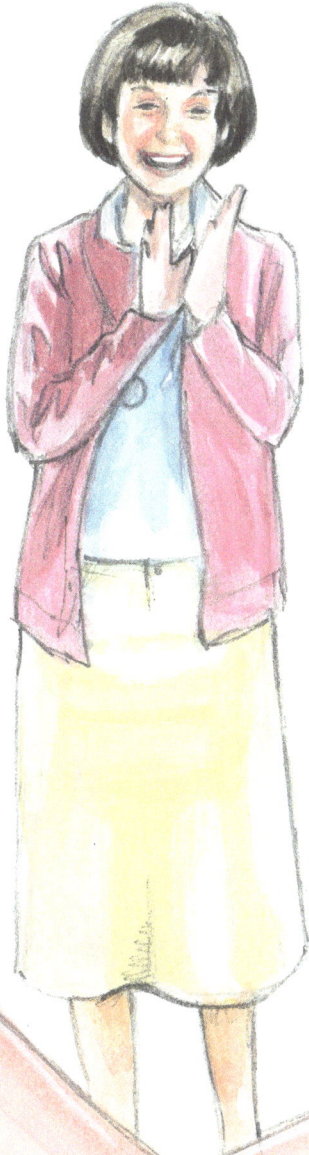
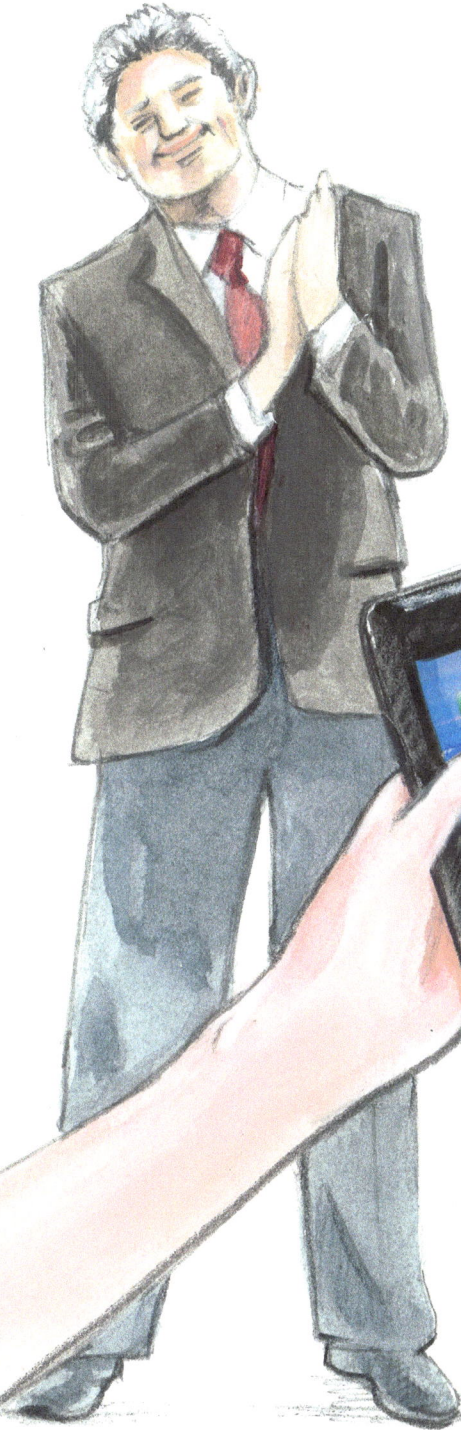
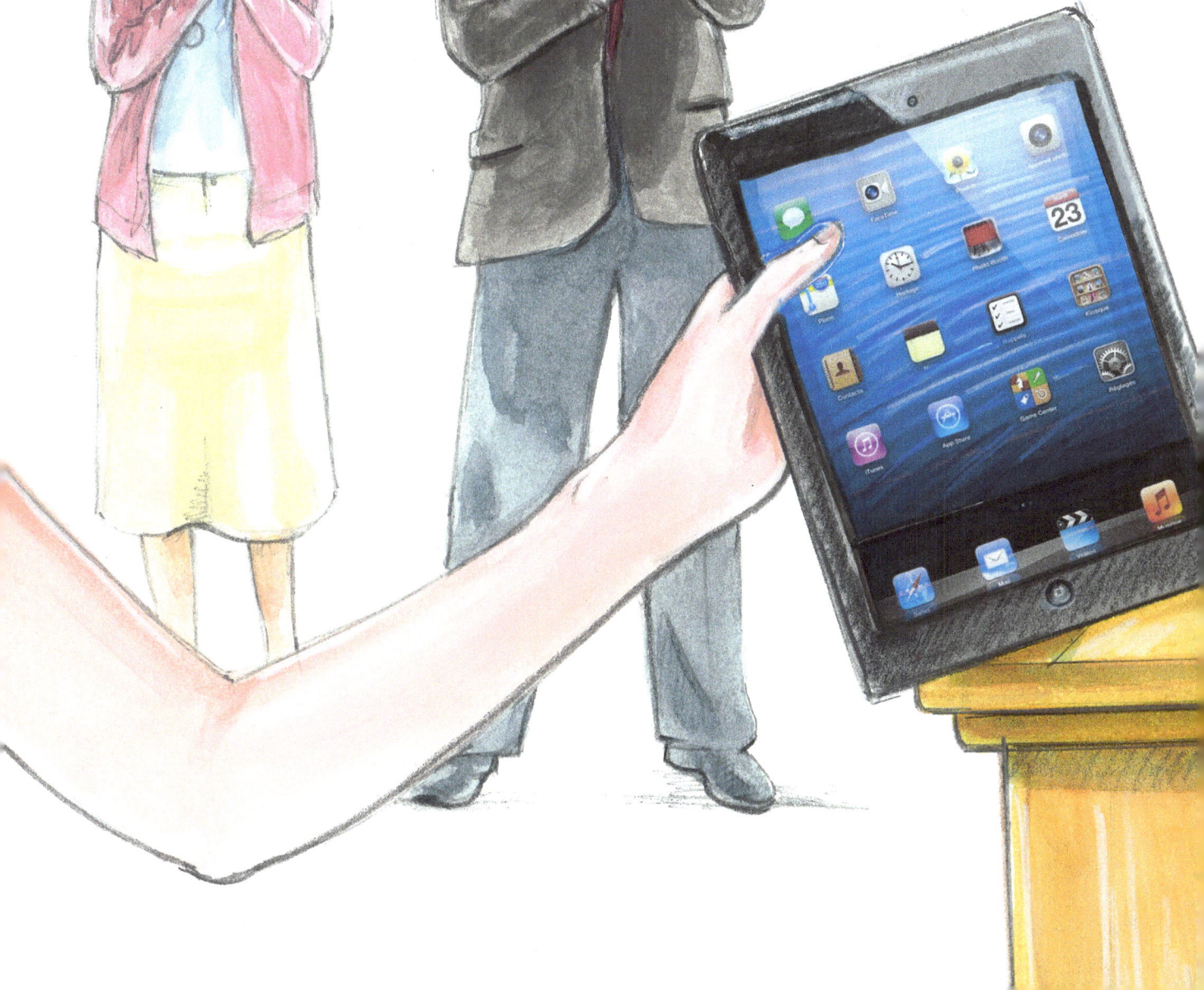

"I am just me."

A Note to Family Members ...

My name is Beverly Burke. I am the proud mother of Sky and four other amazing children.
What you should know is Sky's success did not happen over night. We had many nights crying over homework. Sky woke up most mornings not wanting to go to school and she spent most school days in the nurses' office.

What I want you to know if your child is struggling in school is that it is okay to have them tested. A professional at your school district can do this evaluation or you can do it privately if you choose. This type of assessment should include your child's strengths and weakness. There are lots of strategies that you and your school can use to help your child learn (ex classroom placement, reading programs, writing programs and other types of support service). These assessments may also include recommended accommodations and or modifications like extended time on tests, assistive technology or having a test read to them. If children receive proper services and supports you level their playing field and your child will have greater opportunity for success.

Like Sky I had to learn my rights as her parent and information on her rights to be educated. If you are unsure of your rights call your local Parent or Advocacy center. Speak to other parents whose children receive special education services. You can also do research on the Internet. Sky's Self-Advocacy was inspired by the child friendly website www.imdetermined.org. I'm Determined explained to Sky her significance and role in her education process.

Include your child in his or her educational process. This is their education and they should be a full participant in their process. I used to believe I knew my child best and the services that would fit her best. However, that is not true. Sky knows herself best. She knows what works for her and what doesn't! Learning self-advocacy and understanding her disability and her needs have empowered Sky. Her participation has had a significant positive changed in her education.
Sky believes "You are never to big or small to make a difference in your education".

Being a parent of a child with a disability is not an easy job, as anyone would tell you. An important role we must play is one of a supporter. Remind them everyday of their special qualities. Support your child through the hard times and let them know that even if the special education process is long you will continue until they have the proper supports in school.

One thing I will tell you is not to put all your eggs in one basket. Keep your child engaged in his or her interests.   Your child education is a priority yet they may be struggling eight hours plus, 5 days a week. This can bring anyone down so always expand on and encourage their strengths. Let them explore sports, music, art, technology, or any other interest they may have. This will help them discover who they are and learn that their disability is only one part of their identity. Knowing themselves and being who they are is what will make them a strong and happy individual later on. As long as you believe in your child's full potential everything else will follow!

To get the school to believe in your child's full potential you must believe in your child and his or hers limitless capabilities. In the past school professionals have asked me if I think Sky is lazy? School staff never understood why I wouldn't change her placement to another school outside of our community. The school has stated that Sky is doing well only because she has so many supports and services at school. The school had acted like they never had a child with a Learning Disability in their General education class. In my head and my heart I knew she was not lazy but had a Learning Disability. I knew she belonged in general education with her peers because she is just as smart (maybe even smarter). I knew that when they said she is only doing well because of the supports and services they were saying they finally leveled the playing field for Sky. As her mother I know she wasn't the first student with learning disabilities they had ever had in their class but she definitely is the hardest working, determined student to ever enter their classroom. My belief in Sky, and ultimately her belief in her self transformed the school districts view on her abilities. Now she is a role model to her peers. After many years of hard work the world sees what was always there, a beautiful, intelligent, girl who has many talents and gifts. Sky will, and already is making a big impact in the world.

Respectfully Yours,
Beverly Burke
You can find out more about Sky on her website: theskyislimiless.org

My Spring Vacation
by Sky Burke
April 2011

During my spring vacation I went to Washington D.C. I went to many museums. But my favorite was the Nation History of America. I saw the Ruby Slippers for the Wizard of Oz. Also I saw Kermit the frog from the Muppet Show. We also saw the Lincoln Memorial. You couldn't believe how big it was. But right in front of it was where Martin Luther King Jr. gave his speech. In graved it states: I had a dream by Martin Luther King Jr. If you look straight in the front you would see the reflection pool but it was drained out so was the reflection. I also saw The White House. I saw all the beautiful flowers my favorite was the cherry blossoms. I loved my trip to Washington D.C. I wish I could go again....

Spring Vacation

During spring vacation
I went to Washington D.C.
But I went to many mouses. But
my favorite was the
Natural History of Animals from
I saw the roley also I
the Wizard of Oz.
Saw Cermit the frog some to the
Moris show. We also saw how
Link in Alabama. You could live in
big it was. But right were
point of it. There was his same
Martther King Jr. give his
In grave it sate. I had a
by Mort Ltter King Jr. I saw you
Sijate in frount reflect Shoo
wood see the was and out
port but it was reflection
so the wasing no

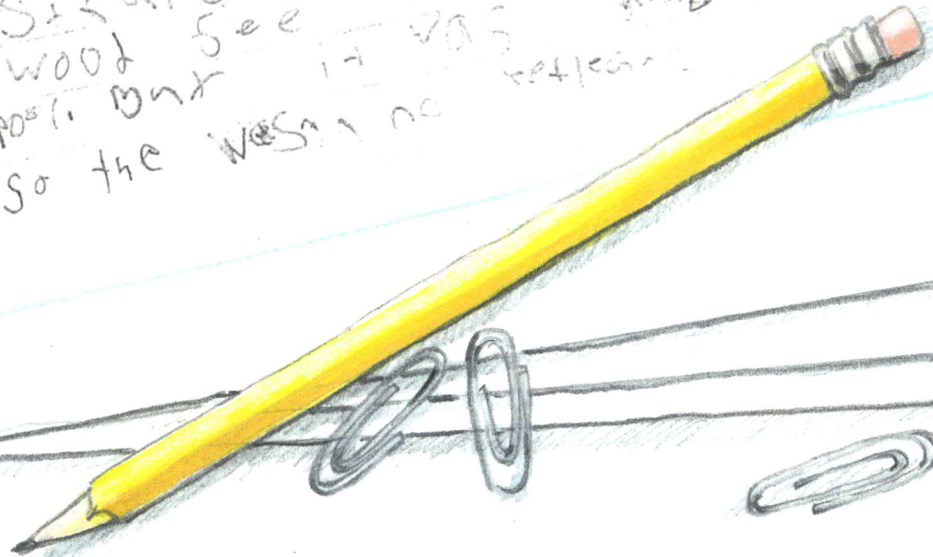

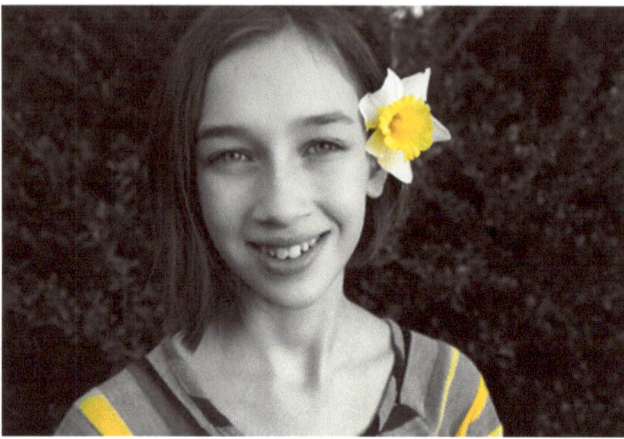

What does a little girl do when she realizes she is different from the other children in her class...when she is being made fun of and isolated because she can't read or write as well as most of her peer group? Since the very beginning of Sky Burke's school experience she had to learn to overcome obstacles and turn lemons into lemonade; Sky had to face challenges and overcome the feeling of being different.

When Sky was four, her dad unexpectedly passed away, leaving her Mom, older sister Aurora and brother Bailey to try to regroup. The healing process was a slow, painful adjustment for her family, especially because they had just moved to a new neighborhood and school several months prior to this life-changing event. As Sky began school, she thought her classmates were learning, reading and writing the same way she did; she thought everyone was having trouble. It was not until the age of seven that she was diagnosed with dyslexia which is difficulty interpreting words and symbols used in reading, as well as dysgraphia, a motor and information processing disability; Sky now knew for sure that she was different from the students in her class. She was emotionally affected by not being able to keep up with the daily school work and having other students not be kind to her; classmates were not interested in being friends with someone who was so "different".

Life changed for Sky when she attended her first CSE meeting with her mom. A CSE meeting is the Committee on Special Education which is usually attended by adults, teachers, specialists and parent(s) of the child. The CSE team wanted to place Sky in a special education class in another school, removing her from her community, siblings and peers. Sky made a decision that she wanted to become an advocate for herself...a self-advocate. This means that she would speak up for herself and let the Committee on Special Education know what she needs; Sky did this! She told the CSE about her special needs over and over again without giving up! Sky created a PowerPoint presentation that demonstrated how technology could help her learn; it showed her strengths and areas that needed to be improved, as well as the role she has played in the school and community around her. She convinced the CSE committee to let her stay in her own school, while getting the proper support. Furthermore, Sky promoted the use of iPads and assisted technology to help other students having the same challenges get the education they deserve.

Today Sky Burke is 12 years old. Sky's family has grown. She has a new dad, Pete and his two daughters, Bailey and Skylar became her sisters. Now there are five siblings with two children named Bailey in their family and a Sky and Skylar, as well! Sky is a passionate reformer, public speaker, and is a driving force that shares her ideas about being a self-advocate through presentations to school administrators, students, teachers, organizations, parents and the business community throughout New York State. Sky dreams of becoming an actress, a lawyer, and the President of the United States.

Sky shares her message, " No Matter How Big or Small You Can Make A BIG Difference!"

The President of The Self-Advocacy Association of NYS Cathy Loquercio Shared These Self-Advocacy Tips With Me.

Speak Up for Yourself- You have a voice use it!

Try, Try again you will get there!

Don't be afraid to ask for help- everybody needs help sometimes!

Trust your own voice-people may not agree with what you want but you still have the right to ask for it.

Talk to people about what you want, talk to people about what you need!

Know your rights- that way no one can take them from you!

Remember you have choices.

Believe in yourself-nobody knows what makes you happiest better than you.

Nothing about me without me!

You have the power to make your own path!

Accept Yourself. Respect Yourself. Love Yourself, Be Yourself!

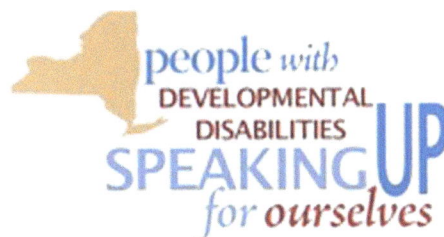

people with
DEVELOPMENTAL
DISABILITIES
SPEAKING UP
for ourselves

Self-Advocacy Association
of New York State, Inc.

www.ingramcontent.com/pod-product-compliance
Lightning Source LLC
LaVergne TN
LVHW072108070426
835509LV00002B/72